A Colour Atlas of
Small Animal Endoscopy

Editors

Malcolm J Brearley

MA, Vet MB, MRCVS

Clinical Oncologist
Animal Health Trust
Newmarket

John E Cooper

BVSc, FRCVS, FIBiol, MRCPath, DTVM

Veterinary Conservator and Senior Lecturer in Comparative Pathology
Royal College of Surgeons of England
London

Martin Sullivan

BVMS, MRCVS, DVR

Lecturer in Soft Tissue Surgery
Department of Veterinary Surgery and Reproduction
University of Glasgow Veterinary School
Glasgow

Wolfe Publishing Limited

Copyright © 1991 Wolfe Publishing Ltd.
Published by Wolfe Publishing Ltd, 1991.
Printed by BPCC Hazell Books Ltd, Aylesbury, England
ISBN 0 7234 1559 5

A CIP catalogue record for this book is available from the British Library.

For a full list of forthcoming titles and details of our surgical, dental and veterinary
atlases, please write to Wolfe Publishing Ltd, 2–16 Torrington Place, London
WC1E 7LT, England.

Contents

Foreword

Recent progress in clinical veterinary medicine, and specifically in the area of diagnostic techniques, has been largely a numbers game. By making use of the ever widening range of laboratory tests conducted on body fluids and tissues, or electromagnetic recordings of bodily activities, we can generate results that allow us to investigate functions of specific body systems very accurately.

These advances may seem to take away the hands-on 'art' of clinical practice. Clinical diagnostic 'art' is the integration of a combination of observations of appearance, feel and responses of the animal to examination. There is only so much that the veterinarian can reach visually or by palpation in an intact animal. As a surgeon, I am well aware of the tremendous advantage that can be obtained by a direct look at, or feel of, tissue, although this often comes at the cost of an involved surgical approach, extended recuperation and the potential for development of complications.

Endoscopy has broadened the application of the 'art' of diagnosis in practice, and permitted the development of a new field of therapeutics. With the newer units and techniques described in this Atlas, orifices and tubular structures can be explored, and sterile body cavities entered in a controlled way that minimises the trauma associated with more invasive techniques.

Now that the technology is readily available, we must accept, as with any clinical procedure, that there is a learning curve associated with its use. Given that our patients require sedation or anaesthesia for endoscopy, there is a particular responsibility to ensure that we obtain the maximum advantage to balance the risks associated with such chemical restraint.

Malcolm Brearley, John Cooper and Martin Sullivan bring very considerable experience to this volume which will help newcomers to endoscopy to become familiar with the appearance of normal and diseased tissues, and encourage them to explore further. For those readers already involved with endoscopy, it will broaden horizons and deepen understanding.

Exotic animal and avian practice often seems to be a peripheral area of clinical veterinary work. However, in the case of endoscopy, those veterinarians engaged in exotic animal practice have been in the forefront of progress because of the special needs of these patients, and the way in which endoscopy can contribute so significantly, as in the sexing of birds.

I have no doubt that new instruments and clinical ingenuity will result in further development of endoscopy in the near future. Some areas with potential, such as arthroscopic surgery, are obvious. Others may be less apparent, but perhaps just as rewarding, for example, equine dentistry, where the long, narrow mouth severely limits visualisation and instrumentation at present.

I welcome this Atlas which will, I believe, be an important contribution to veterinary medicine on both sides of the Atlantic and further afield as well.

Colin E. Harvey, BVSc, FRCVS
Diplomate, American College of Veterinary Surgeons
Diplomate, American Veterinary Dental College
Professor of Surgery
School of Veterinary Medicine
University of Pennsylvania

Preface

" 'The time has come,' the Walrus said, 'to talk of many things . . .' "
Through the Looking Glass, Lewis Carroll
(1832–1898)

Endoscopy has been performed in animals for many years, both for diagnostic and for research purposes. In recent years, however, small animal endoscopy has developed rapidly on account of two unrelated phenomena. First, small animal veterinary practice has gained an increased status proportional to the non-monetary value given by owners to their pets. Secondly, technological developments have brought endoscopic instruments within the budget of the small animal practitioner.

Partially as a result of, and partially in response to, the growth of this investigative technique, a number of excellent texts have been published describing various aspects of endoscopy in pets. However, there is a gap between the scientific papers, with their tendency to describe series of abnormal findings, and the in-depth style of heavyweight textbooks: this Atlas was conceived to fill that void.

In this book we review the major endoscopic techniques that are applicable to small animal veterinary work. Throughout, the emphasis is on the practical aspects and, to that end, contributors with practical experience were sought.

The Atlas is aimed at the practising veterinarian who either has just acquired an endoscope, or is contemplating whether endoscopy might have a place in the practice. It is not intended as a fully comprehensive text, since to cover all techniques that can be, or are, used in small animal endoscopy would require 2–3 times the space available. Equally, no claim is made that the Atlas illustrates every clinical condition that may be encountered. Instead, the Editors draw attention to the value of endoscopy in modern veterinary practice and its potential role in diagnosis and therapy.

In conclusion, the prime objective in compiling this Atlas was to produce a workbook for newcomers to small animal endoscopy and to introduce some of the delights and pitfalls that lie ahead of them!

Malcolm J. Brearley
John E. Cooper
Martin Sullivan

Acknowledgements

The Editors are grateful to all those who have helped in the preparation of this Atlas or provided support and advice. Their thanks are especially due to those who contributed material, without whom the Atlas would not have come to fruition. Professor Colin Harvey very kindly agreed to write the Foreword.

Malcolm Brearley and John Cooper are particularly indebted to Mr Euan Milroy FRCS, Dr Larry Owen and Dr Nina Wedderburn. They helped to establish the Comparative Oncology Unit at the Royal College of Surgeons of England and, in so doing, paved the way for the formulation of the Atlas.

Martin Sullivan wishes to thank Professor G.J. Baker, whose enthusiasm lead to the creation of the veterinary endoscopy service at Glasgow, and to the Royal College of Veterinary Surgeons Spencer-Hill Trust for the further provision of a flexible paediatric bronchoscope.

Special thanks are due to Sally Dowsett for her secretarial assistance, to Frank Sambrook for taking a number of the photographs and to Elaine Penfold for three of the line drawings. The staff of the Royal College of Surgeons and the Royal College of Veterinary Surgeons provided help – and in the case of their libraries, references – on many occasions. Sections of the text were read and commented upon by T.M. Eaton and N. Harcourt-Brown.

The Editors are grateful to the publishers of the following for permission to reproduce illustrations or portions of text in whole or in part:

Journal of Small Animal Practice (British Veterinary Association):

Brearley, M.J. and Cooper, J.E. (1987), **28**, 75–85. The diagnosis of bladder disease in dogs by cystoscopy.

Lindsay, F.E.F. (1983), **24**, 1–15. The normal endoscopic appearance of the caudal reproductive tract of the cyclic and noncyclic bitch: postuterine endoscopy.

Sullivan, M. and Miller, A. (1985), **26**, 369–379. Endoscopy (fibreoptic) of the oesophagus and stomach in the dog with persistent regurgitation or vomiting.

In Practice (British Veterinary Association):

Sullivan, M. (1987), **6**, 217–222. Differential diagnosis of chronic nasal disease in the dog.

The Veterinary Record (British Veterinary Association):

Kivumbi, C.W. and Bennett, D. (1981), **109**, 241–249. Arthroscopy of the canine stifle joint.

Jones, D.M., Samour, J.H., Knight, J.A. and Ffinch, J.M. (1984), **115**, 596–598. Sex determination of monomorphic birds by fibreoptic endoscopy.

Sullivan, M., Lee, R., Fisher, E.W., Nash, A.S.N. and McCandlish, I.A.P. (1987), **120**, 79–83. Gastric carcinoma in the dog: A review of 31 cases.

Blackwell Scientific Publications:

Cooper, J.E. (1988), Rigid endoscopy in exotic species. In *Advances in Small Animal Practice (I)*, (ed) E.A. Chandler.

Finally, thanks are due to the Editors' colleagues and families for their help and encouragement.

List of contributors

The following contributed slides and case histories from which the Editors compiled each chapter:

David Bennett, BSc, BVetMed, PhD, MRCVS, DSAO
Reader in Veterinary Clinical Science, Department of Veterinary Clinical Science, University of Liverpool, PO Box 147, Liverpool L69 3BX, **United Kingdom**
Chapter 10, Canine arthroscopy

Martin Böttcher, Dr med vet
Veterinary Practitioner, PO Box 2164, 5372 Schleiden, **Germany**
Chapter 11, Avian endoscopy

Malcolm J Brearley, MA, Vet MB, MRCVS
Clinical Oncologist, Animal Health Trust, PO Box 5, Newmarket, Suffolk CB8 7DW, **United Kingdom**
Chapter 8, Urethrocystoscopy

John E Cooper, BVSc, FRCVS, FIBiol, MRCPath, DTVM
Veterinary Conservator and Senior Lecturer in Comparative Pathology, Royal College of Surgeons of England, 35–43 Lincoln's Inn Fields, London WC2A 3PN, **United Kingdom**
Chapter 11, Avian endoscopy; Chapter 12, Endoscopy in exotic species

Nigel Harcourt-Brown, BVSc, MRCVS
Practising Veterinary Surgeon, 30 Crab Lane, Bilton, Harrogate, North Yorkshire HG1 3BE, **United Kingdom**
Chapter 11, Avian endoscopy

Brent Jones, DVM
Associate Professor, College of Veterinary Medicine, University of Missouri, Columbia, Missouri 65211, **United States of America**
Chapter 9, Laparoscopy

J Geoffrey Lane, BVetMed, FRCVS
Senior Lecturer, Department of Veterinary Surgery, University of Bristol, Bristol BS18 7DU, **United Kingdom**
Chapter 4, Tracheobronchoscopy

Flora E F Lindsay, MRCVS
(Formerly Senior Lecturer in Veterinary Anatomy, University of Glasgow Veterinary School) Manseburn, Kippen, Stirlingshire FK8 3EF, **United Kingdom**
Chapter 7, Vaginoscopy

Chris May, MA, Vet MB, MRCVS, Cert SAO
Research Fellow, Department of Veterinary Clinical Science, University of Liverpool, PO Box 147, Liverpool L69 3BX, **United Kingdom**
Chapter 10, Canine arthroscopy

Jamie Samour, PhD, MVZ, MIBiol
Al-Areen Wildlife Park, PO Box 28690, **Bahrain**
Chapter 11, Avian endoscopy

Bernd Schildger, Dr med vet
Zoologischer Garten Frankfurt, Alfred-Brehm-Platz 16, 6000 Frankfurt a.M. 1, **Germany**
Chapter 12, Endoscopy in exotic species

Martin Sullivan, BVMS, MRCVS, DVR
Lecturer in Soft Tissue Surgery, Department of Veterinary Surgery and Reproduction, University of Glasgow Veterinary School, Glasgow G61 1QH, **United Kingdom**
Chapter 3, Rhinoscopy; Chapter 4, Tracheobronchoscopy; Chapter 5, Upper alimentary tract endoscopy

David Williams, MA, Vet MB, PhD, MRCVS, DipACVIM
Associate Professor of Medicine, Department of Clinical Sciences, College of Veterinary Medicine, Manhattan, Kansas 66506, **United States of America**
Chapter 6, Lower alimentary tract endoscopy

Tom G Yarrow, BVSc, MRCVS
Practising Veterinary Surgeon, 249/251 Mile End Road, London E1 4BJ, **United Kingdom**
Chapter 9, Laparoscopy

1 Introduction

The term 'endoscopy' is derived from the Ancient Greek, meaning 'to look within'. This is an apt description since modern endoscopic techniques permit internal structures to be examined – and, where appropriate, sampled and treated – with a minimum of distress to, and disturbance of, the patient. As such, they are of value in animals of all ages and health status and can be employed to advantage in non-domesticated, as well as domesticated, species.

The use of endoscopes is not new. There is archaeological evidence that 'vaginal specula' may have been used in Pompeii (Wilbush, 1984 (see Further reading, p.123)) and they were certainly regularly employed in the Middle Ages (Keele, 1963). Two centuries ago, simple instruments were constructed using hollow viewing tubes: a light source was provided using a candle and a mirror (Miller, 1986). Subsequently, the illumination for such basic endoscopes was enhanced by employing oil and gas lamps and, ultimately, electricity. A big advance was the introduction of lenses – either a magnifying eyepiece or several lenses in series. The latter system had many advantages, since it provided a wide field of view, a broad depth of focus, and magnification.

Modern endoscopes, both rigid and flexible, owe their design to the work of Professor Harold Hopkins in the 1950s at Reading University. He developed the 'clad-fibre' system, based upon the earlier work of Baird in the late 1920s. From this came the first truly flexible endoscope. Prior to this, attempts at 'seeing around corners' had depended upon using an array of lenses and prisms; such instruments were cumbersome, had limited mobility and generally gave poorly illuminated images. Fibreoptic bundles revolutionised endoscopy.

The principle of fibreoptics is simple; fine glass fibres are used to transmit light by a process of internal reflection. The clad-fibre system has an inner core of glass with a high refractive index, surrounded by a thin layer of glass with a lower refractive index. This system maximises transmission, with minimal loss of intensity along the length of the fibre. Arranged haphazardly, a bundle of fibres will only transmit light. When aligned such that the array of fibres is an exact match at each end, an image can be faithfully reproduced with relatively little loss of illumination or clarity.

Hopkins also completely transformed rigid endoscopy by introducing his rod lens system. In the first half of the twentieth century, conventional telescope optics of glass lenses with large air gaps were used. The rod lens system utilises glass rods, with precisely ground ends, interspersed by small air spaces. Such systems have minimal problems of spherical and chromatic aberration compared with the conventional lens arrangement.

Microchip electronics have produced the most recent development, in the form of the videoimage endoscope, whereby the optical image is converted into an electrical signal by a solid-state sensor at the distal end of the endoscope. The signal is transmitted by wires up the endoscope, to be interpreted by a computer and displayed on a video monitor.

There have been remarkable advances in endoscopy, but without doubt the technology will continue to progress. Future developments will further increase the versatility of endoscopes and the ability of endoscopists not only to investigate and to diagnose, but also to treat their patients by minimally invasive techniques.

In this Atlas the use of endoscopy in small animals, including 'exotic' species, is outlined and pictorial examples are given of normal and abnormal structures.

There are two main approaches to endoscopic examination:

- Via a natural orifice, as in tracheoscopy and gastroscopy.
- Via an artificial aperture, as in arthroscopy and laparoscopy.

Both approaches are covered in this volume.

Endoscopes are still relatively expensive, but they have so much to commend them. They provide opportunities to investigate and study normal and abnormal organs and tissues in a wide range of species. The techniques used are relatively non-invasive and thus not only particularly appropriate to aged or debilitated patients but also, since the amount of surgery required is usually minimal and anaesthesia only light, highly acceptable on welfare grounds. There are generally few postoperative complications and rarely any need for concern over the 'cosmetic' effects of the procedure.

Endoscopy is a truly multidisciplinary subject that concerns not only those in the medical and veterinary fields: without physicists and engineers the instrumentation would not exist in its present form. Clinicians, including general physicians, general surgeons and specialists in many fields, form the majority of those who employ endoscopy. However, non-clinicians, such as pathologists and microbiologists, often rely upon endoscopy to provide good quality specimens for diagnosis. Endoscopy of animals is not only important in its own right but can also play a part in biomedical research and the development of new procedures.

Endoscopy is an art, as well as a science, and techniques can only be learned as a result of practical tuition and experience. Nevertheless, part of the skill of the endoscopist is in distinguishing abnormality from normality and in interpreting changes in organs and tissues. This Atlas aims to help achieve this.

2 The endoscope – practical considerations

Choice of endoscope

In small animal practice it is difficult to justify the purchase of a full range of endoscopes because of budgetary constraints. The choice between a rigid or flexible endoscope is usually determined by the procedures to be performed, but there are a number of points to consider: the main areas in which the endoscope is to be deployed, the range of animal sizes likely to be dealt with, and any samples that are to be collected.

Rigid endoscopes

Rigid endoscopes tend to be designed for one technique only; however, it is worth considering those additional procedures the instrument could be put to, given minor modifications. The smaller manufacturers of endoscopes may be amenable to modifying existing instruments, on request, at a reasonable cost. For example, by supplying both a blunt-ended obturator and a sharp trocar with a laparoscope, this one instrument can be used not only for cystoscopy and laparoscopy in mammals and birds, but also for rhinoscopy in larger dogs and rigid tracheoscopy in mammals, birds and reptiles.

Flexible endoscopes

In general practice the two areas in which the flexible endoscope is mainly used are the lower respiratory tract and the gastrointestinal tract. These regions require an endoscope that is reasonably narrow and at least 1 m long. It must have an irrigation and insufflation facility to allow the objective lens to be washed and the alimentary tract to be filled with air. A sampling channel that permits the taking of brushings, biopsies and aspirates is very useful. However, the external diameter requirements place a constraint on the diameter of the sampling channel and, therefore, on the size and the depth of the biopsies.

For the oesophagus, stomach, trachea, bronchi and vagina, a forward-viewing (panendoscope) endoscope is most satisfactory. The above requirements are best met by a paediatric gastroscope of 9 mm diameter and 1 m working length. However, its diameter and working length may prevent it from being used successfully to examine the duodenum of small and giant breeds of dogs. It can also be used for tracheobronchoscopy of dogs weighing more than 10 kg, but care must be taken to ensure adequate oxygenation, and to avoid asphyxiating the animal by over-enthusiastic endoscopic observation.

Second-hand equipment

It is often possible to obtain second-hand equipment from human hospitals. Such equipment may seem like a bargain, but one should be aware that the cost of repairing or servicing this type of endoscope can be very great. In considering a purchase, care should be taken to ensure that an existing light source is compatible, or that one is available at reasonable cost. In general, 150 W tungsten light sources are cheaper to run than xenon light sources.

Potential purchases should always be examined with a light source attached. This is to check that an excessive number of fibre bundles are not broken (one of the major reasons for hospitals discarding endoscopes). Endoscopes with more than 10–15% of the bundles broken should not be purchased. The bending angles should be tested. It is inevitable that the control wires stretch, so reducing the range of bending. The insertion tube should be checked for damage and the seals for evidence of wear and leaks. The irrigation and insufflation controls must be working, and the light source, which usually contains the pumps, must have leads that fit the light guide connector.

Battery-powered endoscopes

Battery-powered endoscopes, including modified auriscopes (otoscopes), have much to commend them. They are a useful first step for the practitioner who requires a relatively inexpensive kit for endoscopic examination of domesticated and 'exotic' species. In addition – and perhaps more importantly – they have the advantage of being lightweight and, since they are independent of an external power source, they can be easily taken on house calls or into the field. Just as rigid and flexible endoscopes are looked upon as complementary to one another, a battery-operated instrument should be considered a necessary part of the veterinary endoscopist's armoury.

Basic care of endoscopes

Modern endoscopes are delicate and expensive instruments. Since the major component of both flexible and rigid endoscopes is glass, the instrument should be treated in a suitable manner. With careful handling and use, an endoscope may have a prolonged life.

Storage

Rigid endoscopes are best stored and transported in rigid boxes with foam inserts (1). This prevents bending and jarring of these delicate instruments.

Flexible instruments may be transported in a similar manner to avoid sharp knocks in transit, which can cause fibre bundle breakage. However, they are best stored in a hanging position, preferably in a secure cabinet. This prevents permanent curvature developing and permits water to drain out of the various channels in the insertion tube.

All endoscopes are best stored at normal room temperature and relative humidity; extremes and marked variations of either may be deleterious Endoscopes that have been stored in a cold room, or transported in the luggage compartment of a car during winter, should be allowed to warm to room temperature before use; at low temperatures the glass elements become more brittle and are more liable to break.

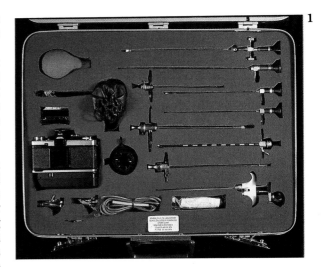

1 Rigid endoscopes in their transport case.

Disinfection and sterilisation

When performing endoscopic procedures, infection and contamination of the system being examined must be minimised. Aseptic technique should be performed wherever possible, although the degree of stringency can be reduced in certain cases, for example, for colonoscopy. The manufacturers' recommendations regarding cleaning and disinfection should be observed for individual instruments. The comments that follow are very general guidelines.

Flexible fibreoptic and rigid glass telescope endoscopes **should not** be heat sterilised (dry oven or autoclave), unless specifically advocated by the manufacturers. For these delicate instruments, some form of chemical sterilisation or disinfection should be used. Where available, ethylene oxide gas is the disinfectant of choice for arthroscopes and laparoscopes. However, submersion in activated glutaraldehyde solution (Cidex™, Johnson and Johnson, UK) is a more convenient method for routine disinfection and, given sufficient time, sterilisation of most endoscopes. Although the new generation flexible fibrescopes are fully immersible, care should be exercised with older models in order to prevent water entering and damaging the internal structures of the instrument.

It should be remembered that glutaraldehyde is an excellent fixative. If the endoscope is not rinsed prior to use, body tissues may be damaged. Likewise, if the instruments are not washed after a procedure, blood and other body fluids that accumulate on the objective lens or in the irrigation channel may be fixed. Subsequent cleaning can prove difficult and damage may occur.

Personal protection

It is good practice to wear sterile gloves when performing endoscopy. Not only does this protect the animal from contamination, but it also protects the clinician. Further precautions should be taken in special circumstances. A facemask and goggles should be considered when performing upper airway endoscopy in dogs or birds in which the zoonoses tuberculosis or chlamydiosis are a potential danger. Great care should be taken with primates, in which tuberculosis and, especially *Herpesvirus simiae* (B-virus) may be present (see Chapter 12). The use of teaching heads or a camera and monitor can reduce the health risk to the endoscopist.

Basic use

- Rigid telescopes should be picked up by the eyepiece and **not** by the rod.
- Flexible endoscopes should be carried by the control section, with the insertion tube supported by the other hand to prevent trailing and damage to the distal end.
- Rigid telescopes should never be bent, even a few degrees. At the very least this may permanently distort the light path; more seriously, it will crack a glass section. The use of cannulae or rigid sheaths may protect the telescope from bending forces.
- Flexible fibrescopes should not be subjected to a curvature of less than 2 cm radius. Beyond this, fibres may be broken and guide wires stretched, rendering the instrument unserviceable.
- Care should be taken not to knock or drop the instruments.

Problems encountered during viewing

Smears on objective lens

Body fluids and, in particular, blood on the objective lens will hamper vision (**2**). In some endoscopes the irrigation channel is arranged so that it flushes across the objective. Where this facility is not available, it may be necessary to withdraw the endoscope completely and wipe the lens clean with soft lens tissue paper. During laparoscopy, smears may sometimes be cleared by pressing the objective against the mesentery and gently rotating the endoscope prior to redirection. A bowl of warm saline is of value for washing the tip of the instrument.

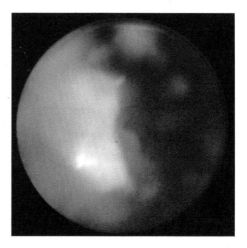

2 Smears on objective lens. Smeared mucus is covering part of the lens and obscuring the lesion of interest – a fungal plaque in the nasal cavity. Note the blurring and chromatic aberration.

Fogging

The temperature difference between the optical parts of an endoscope and the internal cavity of the animal may be in excess of 10°C; as a result, water vapour will condense on the objective lens. Similarly, condensation may occur on the eyepiece from water vapour in the endoscopist's breath (this is exacerbated when the operator is wearing a facemask). Anti-fogging agents are commercially available and can be applied to the eyepiece and objective lenses before use. Alternatively, the endoscope can be placed in an incubator or water-bath to warm the instruments to body temperature.

'Red-out'

'Red-out' is the colloquial term for the view that is obtained when the objective is pushed up against tissue. The redness is due to the diffuse, red glow that is seen when tissues are transilluminated. Withdrawal and redirection, or increased distension of a hollow organ, should correct this problem.

Overinsufflation

Overinsufflation (**3**) can cause hollow organs (e.g., stomach) to mould against adjacent solid structures (e.g., liver) creating the impression of a submucosal or intramural mass.

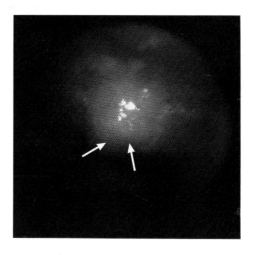

3 Overinsufflation. In this endoscopic view of a dog with megaoesophagus, the bony protuberances of the cervical vertebrae can be seen to impinge (arrows) on the oesophageal lumen, mimicking mural masses. This view also illustrates the problem of poor illumination of a large, hollow structure: poor light reflection can make tissues appear darker than they actually are.

Poor illumination

Poor illumination may be due to a number of problems:

- A damaged light guide.
- Failing batteries (where applicable).
- Smears of blood etc on illumination lenses.
- Overdistension of a hollow organ taking the object of interest out of the range of illumination.

Turbidity of the viewing medium

Turbidity (4) is only a problem when viewing through a fluid, as in urethrocystoscopy or arthroscopy. Turbidity may be caused by cellular debris or bleeding. Further irrigation and fresh saline should improve the clarity.

Biopsies or endoscopy surgery should only be attempted once a complete examination of the cavity has been performed; otherwise turbidity may result.

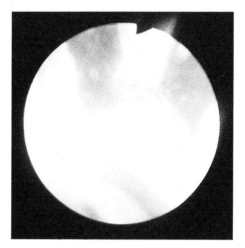

4

4 Turbidity of the viewing medium. Saline is used in urethrocystoscopy to distend the bladder and act as the viewing medium. Here, the reflection from suspended particulate matter all but obliterates the view of a papillary tumour.

Glare and reflection

Bubbles over the end of the endoscope cause serious distortion of vision (5). Likewise, reflection from serous surfaces can mask adjacent or underlying lesions. In avian laparoscopy the air sacs will reflect the light, but if the objective is moved closer, the light will shine through and structures on the other side will be seen.

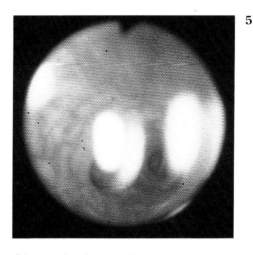

5

5 Glare and reflection. A bubble from fluid flushed across the lens reflects the light transmitted down the twin light guides of a flexible endoscope.

Iatrogenic lesions

Care should be taken not to damage tissues with the tip of the endoscope (**6**); although only minor injury is usually caused, the defect may mimic pathological lesions. In the stomach, for example, such iatrogenic lesions may be mistaken for small ulcers by the inexperienced.

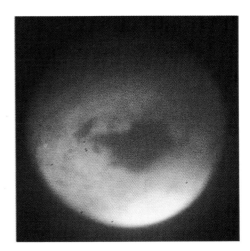

6 Iatrogenic lesions. Iatrogenic mucosal erosion and haemorrhage may be caused by pushing the endoscope blindly on to the greater curvature of the stomach wall, and may mimic small ulcers.

Artefacts due to endoscope problems

Broken fibres

Broken fibres (**7**) are seen as black dots across the image, and arise through mishandling and rough use of the endoscope. A row of broken fibres suggests excessive bending in one plane.

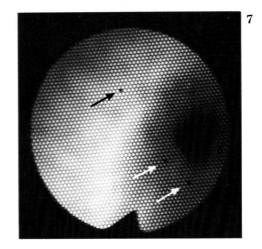

7 Broken fibres. Although the hexagonal array of the fibres of a flexible endoscope cannot be avoided, the replacement of individual fibres by black dots (arrows) should be: each represents a broken fibre.

Browning

A brown hue to the image is highly suggestive of water having leaked into the system via the various seals. Many modern flexible instruments have a facility for leakage testing which can alert the user to a problem at an early stage and the need for repair.

Eclipsing

Eclipsing (**8**) occurs when the telescope has been bent such that an image of the telescope wall is seen as a crescent. This artefact indicates a serious fault in the handling of a rigid telescope. It can break the glass rods of the instrument.

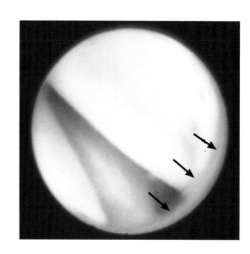

8

8 Eclipsing. This is a problem seen with rigid glass rod type telescopes. It occurs when a bending moment applied to the telescope takes the lens system out of true alignment, and can lead to a glass segment snapping. Note the crescent (arrows) at the edge of the field.

Teaching aids, records and photography

Teaching attachments are useful adjuncts to endoscopic examination. These can be of rigid or flexible construction, and with a 'C' mount, some small inexpensive videocameras can be attached. They allow a second person to view the examination and can thus be used for teaching and also for second opinions.

Records are an important part of endoscopy because the examination does not provide a single photographic image, as would radiography, but constitutes the visualisation in the examiner's mind of the topography of the organ(s) through the build-up of many images. These are easily forgotten and it is necessary to make a permanent record. This record most usefully takes the form of a written report, combined with photographic or videoimages. These allow comparison during serial examinations and also provide illustrative and teaching material.

Endoscopic photography requires a high intensity light, preferably with flash facilities and special mounts to couple the camera to the eyepiece of the endoscope. In the absence of photography, drawings are of value. It may be useful to have duplicated record sheets with a stylised outline drawing of the structure in question: lesions and abnormal findings can be superimposed at the time of the examination.

3 Rhinoscopy

Introduction

Rhinoscopy is indicated for the investigation of a range of clinical signs including nasal discharge, sneezing, epistaxis, and rhinarial ulceration. It is particularly useful for differentiating between neoplasia, aspergillosis, foreign body, chronic hyperplastic rhinitis and other forms of destructive rhinitis.

Choice of instrument

Rhinoscopy can be divided into rostral and caudal rhinoscopy. Rostral examinations can be performed with a variety of instruments including flexible and rigid paediatric bronchoscopes, arthroscopes, and otoscopes (auriscopes) with long specula. Caudal rhinoscopy requires the use of a flexible endoscope or a bright light source and a dental mirror.

Technique

Preparation

Since the nasal cavity is particularly sensitive, the choice of anaesthetic technique is important: muscle relaxants and artificial ventilation, or additional analgesia with local anaesthetic spray, or high-dose opiate analgesics may be necessary to reduce movement or sneezing. A dog or cat is best positioned on its chest, with the nose close to the edge of the table, thus allowing the endoscopist to examine both sides in comfort, and negating the need to turn the patient. Any visible discharge in the nasal vestibule should be removed to clear the opening, so that it does not smear the objective lens. Excessive discharge and induced haemorrhage are often encountered in rhinoscopy and cannot be reduced by careful preparation.

Insertion

Rostrally, the endoscope has to be guided past the lateral wing of the nostril by inserting the end of the instrument in a dorsal and medial direction, then swinging the body of the endoscope medially, thus displacing the lateral cartilage and allowing the endoscope to be advanced into the common meatus. Caudally, a flexible endoscope can be passed into the laryngopharynx and then hooked over the soft palate. The alternative, a warmed dental mirror, is placed caudal to the soft palate, which has been drawn forwards with a hook or forceps, so that the light is reflected into the nasopharynx.

Orientation and examination

Orientation and examination can best be achieved by identifying the nasal septum and the meatus rostrally, and the choanae when caudal rhinoscopy is performed.

Problems encountered during rhinoscopy are associated with discharge and haemorrhage (pre-existing and induced) severely limiting vision. Full examination of the turbinate scrolls is not possible owing to their shape and complexity. The base of the maxilloturbinates may also restrict further passage caudally to the ethmoturbinates.

Despite these problems, rhinoscopy is a quick procedure and one that can be performed following radio-logical investigation. Examination can be rewarding in some cases of neoplasia, although the appearance of chronic hyperplastic rhinitis and neoplasia may be indistinguishable. Rhinoscopy comes into its own for the investigation of destructive rhinitis, since radiology cannot distinguish between mycotic and non-mycotic destructive rhinitis. Obstruction of the nasal passages due to a foreign body may be difficult to diagnose radiologically, as frequently the object is radiolucent and causes little turbinate damage; in many cases, rhinoscopy not only provides the diagnosis, but also the treatment.

Normal appearance

Rostral view

9

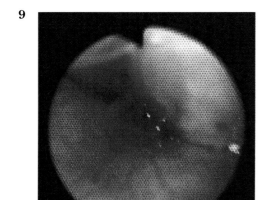

9 Rostral view. The endoscope pushes the turbinates apart as it is advanced along the common meatus. The red blush to parts of the mucosa is easily caused by impingement of the instrument on the sensitive nasal mucosa.

10

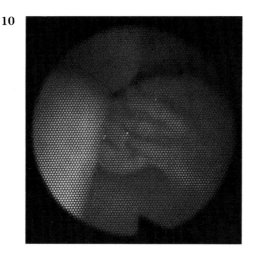

10 Rostral view. The root of the maxilloturbinates is visible only in large breeds of dogs, and in those where the rostrally situated scrolls have been destroyed. The colour of the mucosa is variable, depending on the proximity of the endoscope to the mucosa, and the angle at which the transmitted light is reflected.

11 Rostral view. The nasal septum appears much paler than the turbinates, but has a distinct interlacing network of vessels.

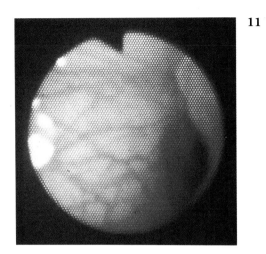

Nasopharynx

12 Nasopharynx. In this view the openings of the Eustachian tubes are visible as small, white, raised areas. The whiteness is due to reflection. The caudal choanae are not visible, since the endoscope has not been advanced far enough rostrally.

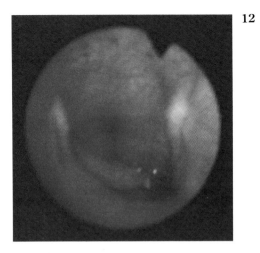

13 Nasopharynx. The mucosa should be a pale pink, with obvious but fine blood vessels coursing submucosally. The caudal choanae should be just visible in the distance, but this depends on the intensity of the light source and the length of the soft palate. There should be no discharge present.

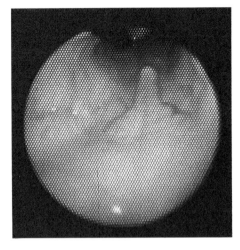

Abnormal appearance

Neoplasia

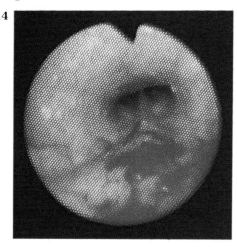

14   Neoplasia. In this view of the nasopharynx the caudal choanae are visible, and fresh blood may be seen flowing from both nasal chambers. (A ten-year-old Yorkshire terrier with bilateral nasal discharge, occasional epistaxis and absent airflow.)

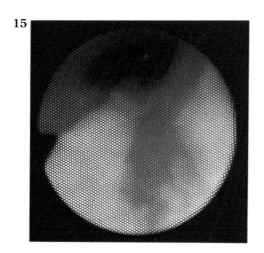

15   Neoplasia. Caudal rhinoscopy demonstrates a pool of clotted blood. It is not possible to determine the site of origin, as the soft palate was too long to allow the endoscope to be pulled far enough forwards, but the blood is lying to the right side. (A six-year-old Labrador with daily nose bleeds and a reduced airflow.)

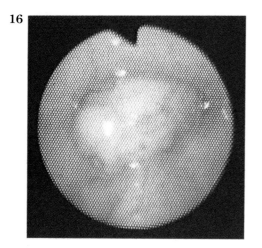

16   Neoplasia. Using caudal rhinoscopy, a large, pale, firm mass is seen occluding the nasopharynx. The tentative diagnosis of non-lymphoid neoplasia in a 12-year-old, mouth-breathing cat was confirmed histopathologically as an adeno-carcinoma.

17   Neoplasia. Rostral rhinoscopy demonstrates a small,
red mass protruding from the middle meatus into the
common meatus. During endoscopy, the area quickly
haemorrhaged and a red stream enveloped the end-piece.
As no conclusive diagnosis could be reached, a rhinotomy
and turbinectomy had to be performed and the submitted
tissue was found to be neoplastic. Induced haemorrhage is
an example of a problem that bedevils good endoscopic
examination of nasal tumours.

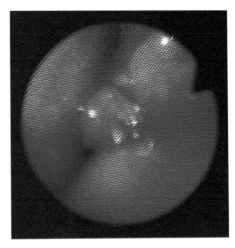

17

18   Neoplasia. Using rostral rhinoscopy, a mass can be
seen pushing the turbinates apart. Through the surface of
the mass a number of small blood vessels are visible. The
mass is distinguishable from a turbinate only because it is
pushing the true turbinates apart.

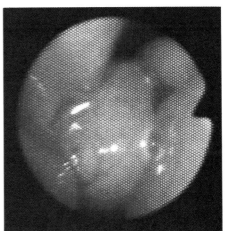

18

19   Neoplasia. The left nasal chamber shows a bulging of
the septum into the common meatus, and a large, irregular-
surfaced, pink mass occupying the ventral part of the
common meatus. Following the introduction of the endoscope
into the right nostril, only haemorrhage was visible. (A nine-
year-old Labrador with right mucopurulent nasal discharge,
and radiographic evidence of septal destruction.)

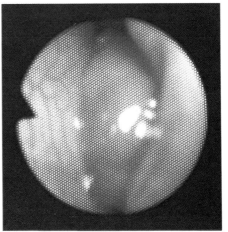

19

23

Chronic hyperplastic rhinitis

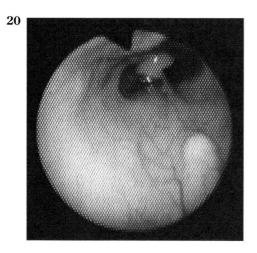

20 Chronic hyperplastic rhinitis. At caudal rhinoscopy, the mucosa of the nasopharynx is normal, but there is a bead of mucopus dorso-laterally. In the distance, a globule of mucopus is visible on the septum, between the caudal choanae.

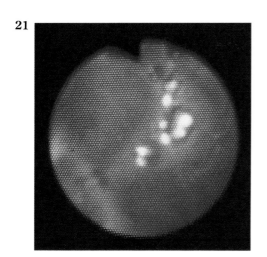

21 Chronic hyperplastic rhinitis. Rostrally, the turbinates are inflamed; the air channels are not visible as they are occluded by a green discharge. (A four-year-old cross-bred dog with unilateral purulent discharge of four months' duration.)

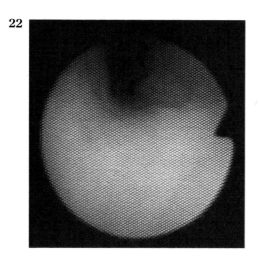

22 Chronic hyperplastic rhinitis. The nasopharynx is clouded in a river of purulent material, obscuring the normal blood vessel pattern. (A six-year-old dachshund with persistent bilateral discharge, partially responsive to antibiotics and bromhexine hydrochloride.)

Aspergillosis

23 Aspergillosis. There is a relatively dry lesion, absence of discharge and a loss of turbinates, which would normally have blocked the passage of the endoscope to the ethmoturbinates. There is a large fungal plaque with a green speckled appearance and to one side there is a dark mass of clotted blood. (A three-year-old golden retriever with a 14-day history of intermittent bouts of unilateral epistaxis and a slight green discharge, with difficulty prehending food. There was rhinarial swelling, ulceration and depigmentation, and the dog resented palpation of the nose.)

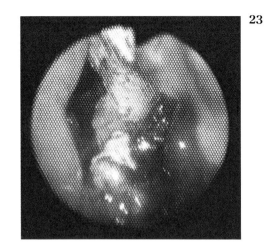

23

24 Aspergillosis. There is a mucoid discharge in the ventral meatus apparently confluent with a brilliant-white, dry, fungal plaque. Note the lack of turbinate scrolls. (A two-year-old German shepherd dog with purulent nasal discharge, inappetence and facial pain.)

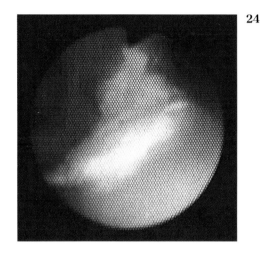

24

25 Aspergillosis. A large dirty yellow mass, with a central cleavage line, lies 6 cm from the nares. This was removed and found to be a fungal ball or aspergilloma lying in an otherwise empty nasal cavity. (A seven-year-old Labrador with a 12-month history of frequent but intermittent nasal discharge, responsive to a variety of antibiotics.)

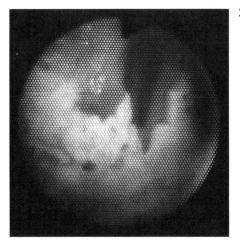

25

26

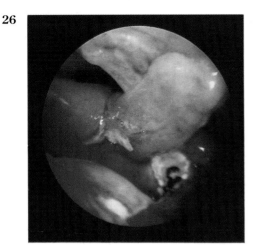

27

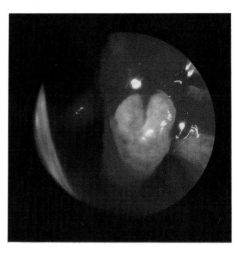

26 & 27 A small fungal plaque with a black centre is present on the turbinates. A truncated turbinate is swollen with further plaques on abutting mucosa. Following treatment with ketoconazole, the fungal plaques have disappeared and the truncated turbinate has shrunk. Haemorrhage has been induced by the endoscope.

28

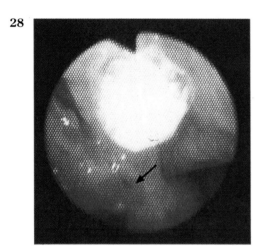

28 A small white fungal plaque is visible adjacent to the drainage ostium (arrow) of the frontal sinus, four weeks post-surgery, in a four-year-old Staffordshire bull terrier that was unsuccessfully treated twice with chemotherapy. The infection eventually resolved.

29

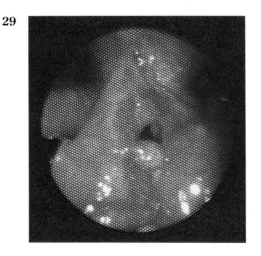

29 One month post-enilconazole treatment. The widened frontal sinus ostium (centre field), through which a drain had been implanted, is visible surrounded by mucosa that is still somewhat inflamed.

30 One month post-enilconazole treatment. A lack of turbinates is noted and the nasopharynx is visible in the distance. The remaining turbinates are irregular and knobbly.

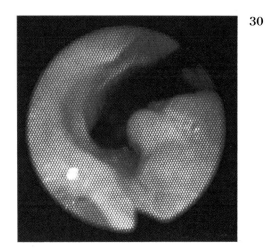

30

31 Six months post-treatment. A large, irregular area of turbinate is present at the base of the residual maxilloturbinates. This an attempt by the turbinate to regenerate.

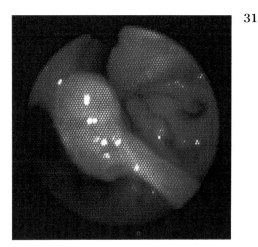

31

32 One month post-treatment. The dog had responded quickly to treatment and the drainage hole in the frontal bone had healed quickly. A small, glistening mass (1 mm across) is seen in the frontal sinus. When grasped with forceps and removed, it proved to be a small fragment of bone, thought to have arisen from the creation of the drain hole in the frontal bone.

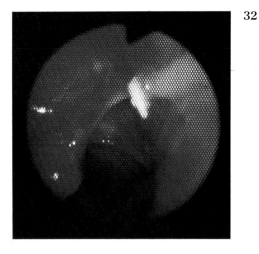

32

Foreign body

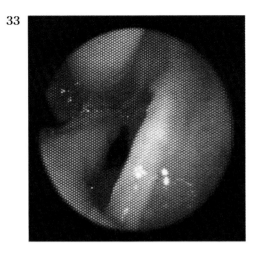

33 **Foreign body.** A stick covered in yellow mucus can be seen running between the turbinates caudally. (A two-year-old springer spaniel working dog which had emerged from some undergrowth in a frenzy of sneezing with slight epistaxis.)

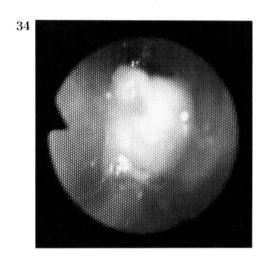

34 **Foreign body.** A twig, seen end-on, is surrounded by inflamed and swollen turbinates which have wedged the twig in place. There is also some purulent material.

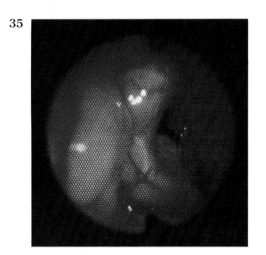

35 **Foreign body.** The same case as in **34**, following removal of the twig. A curved impression caused by the lodged twig is visible in the turbinate facing the septum.

36   Foreign body. Rostral view. A four-year-old German shepherd dog presented with rhinarial ulceration and a slight nasal discharge of six weeks' duration. Under anaesthesia, a small hole was found in the alar fold. A needle, seen lying between the turbinates, was pulled through the defect in the alar fold.

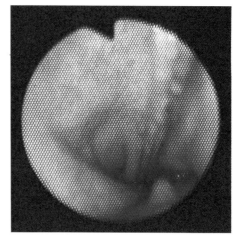

37   Foreign body. A thick blade of grass, 6 cm long, sits in the nasopharynx, extending forwards into the nasal cavity. (A six-year-old, domestic short-haired cat with a bilateral nasal discharge, persistent sneezing and upper respiratory noise had been unresponsive to a variety of antibiotics given over a three-month period.)

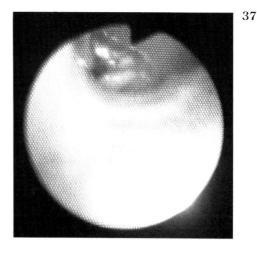

Polyp

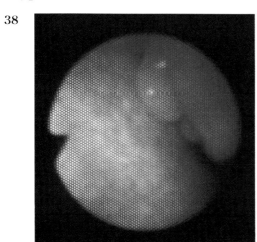

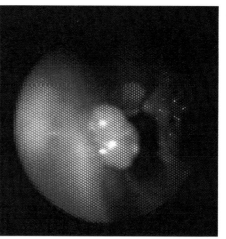

38   Polyp. A small pink mass is seen pushing between the septum and the turbinates. This could easily be due to neoplastic tissue, and biopsy is required to confirm the diagnosis. (A four-year-old Labrador presented with intermittent epistaxis of one month duration.)

39   Polyp. The same dog as shown in **38** three months post-rhinotomy. There is an absence of turbinates, but on the lateral wall there is a small, irregular, regenerating turbinate.

Idiopathic destructive rhinitis

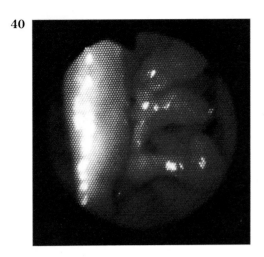

40 Idiopathic destructive rhinitis. Truncated turbinates are present in a two-year-old English pointer with mucopurulent nasal discharge, but no facial pain or reduction in airflow. The dog was serologically negative for *Aspergillus* and *Penicillium* species.

4 Tracheobronchoscopy

Introduction

The principle indications for tracheobronchoscopy are respiratory stridor or coughing, for which there are many causes including trauma, tracheobronchitis, tracheal collapse, parasitic infestation, foreign body obstruction and neoplasia. Endoscopy is important in the identification and removal of tracheal and bronchial foreign bodies, although difficulties with anaesthesia may necessitate repeated attempts at removal.

Severe dyspnoea due to pulmonary pathology is a major contraindication. Endoscopy should be avoided in those cases in which there is evidence of acute upper respiratory infection. Although rare in dogs, pulmonary tuberculosis is a cause of chronic coughing, and owing to its zoonotic potential, proper personal precautions (e.g., goggles and facemask) should be taken for **all** upper airway endoscopic procedures. Tuberculosis highlights the need for proper evaluation of the patient (including radiography) before undertaking endoscopy.

Choice of instrument

Both rigid and flexible instruments can be used for tracheobronchoscopy. However, rigid instruments are effectively limited to the first generation bronchi, whereas flexible endoscopes can be steered down and around the bronchial divisions, the only limiting factor being the diameter of the endoscope relative to the bronchus. Because of the variability in the size of dogs a selection of bronchoscopes is required to examine all breeds. A paediatric bronchoscope is excellent for the small dog and cat, and a paediatric gastroscope can double as a bronchoscope for the larger breeds. Apart from visual examination, samples for microbiological, parasitological and cytological examination are needed for a complete evaluation of the patient; thus, the bronchoscope requires a channel for aspiration, biopsy forceps and cytology brushes.

Technique

Preparation

Standard withholding times for food and fluids are satisfactory. Premedication with atropine should be avoided as it suppresses secretion in the respiratory tract. The length of the anticipated examination and local routine determines the choice of induction agent. Although the animal can be positioned in dorsal recumbency, ventral recumbency permits easier orientation and identification of the bronchial divisions. The main consideration during bronchoscopy is maintenance of the airway. Care should be taken to ensure oxygenation by observing the colour of the mucous membranes and by supplying oxygen through the endoscope or via a thin tube running parallel to the endoscope.

Insertion

The endoscope may be introduced through the larynx or down the lumen of the endotracheal tube. Care should be taken to avoid the teeth when the endoscope is introduced *per os*. It is frequently easier to pass the endoscope over the epiglottis and through the larynx with the naked eye, rather than using the optics of the endoscope. The trachea and bronchi are best examined after induction of anaesthesia.

Orientation

The tracheal ligament allows the dorsum of the trachea to be identified. At the bifurcation of the trachea, the carina presents as a sharp pillar. The right bronchus is that nearly in line with the trachea, whereas the left bronchus is set at an angle. On the right, bronchi are given off in the following order: cranial lobe (laterally), middle lobe (ventrally), accessory lobe (ventromedially) and finally, the caudal lobe. The major divisions on the left are to the cranial lobe (ventrolaterally) and the caudal lobe. From each of these bronchi a variable number of segmental divisions arise.

Normal endoscopic appearance

Normal trachea

41

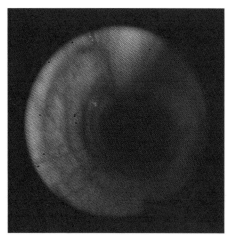

41 Normal appearance. The mucous membrane is a pale, pink-yellow colour, with an obvious vascular pattern. The C-shaped tracheal rings create marked indentations in the mucous membrane. Between the arms of the tracheal rings, the tracheal ligament can be seen running the length of the trachea as a strap-like fold of tissue. The trachea is widest at the point where it joins the larynx. In the normal animal, no material is present in the trachea or main stem bronchi.

Abnormal endoscopic appearance

Laryngeal oedema

42

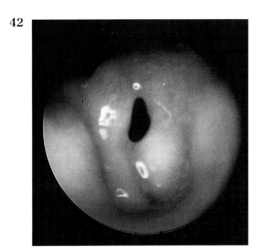

42 Laryngeal oedema. The larynx of the cat can respond in a rapid and marked fashion to trauma, whether from foreign body stimulation or iatrogenically from rough endotracheal intubations. Oedema and inflammation can cause sufficient swelling of the vocal cords and mucosa of the arytenoid cartilages to compromise severely the rima glottidis.

Tracheobronchitis

43 Tracheobronchitis. The mucous membrane of the trachea and the main stem bronchi are red and inflamed. Globules of mucopus are present along the length of the tract, and the fold of mucous membrane associated with the dorsal tracheal ligament is widened and thickened at the bifurcation. The swelling of the mucous membrane may result in some narrowing of the lumen of the bronchi. (A two-year-old greyhound with a persistent cough of three weeks' duration, accompanied by reduced performance.)

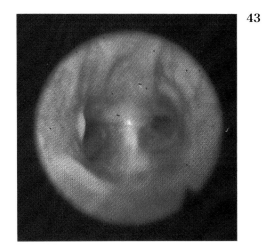

43

Tracheal collapse

44

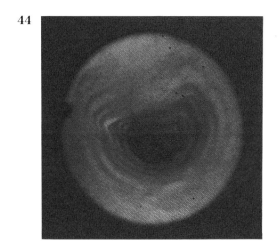

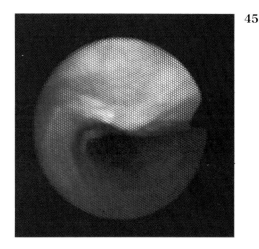

45

44 Tracheal collapse. Throughout the cervical trachea the strap-like fold of mucous membrane is absent and the tips of the tracheal rings are widely separated with a flat membrane, which moved with respiration. Diagnosis: tracheal collapse exacerbated by cardiorespiratory disease in an eight-year-old obese cavalier King Charles spaniel.

45 Tracheal collapse. The tracheal rings are D-shaped, the tracheal ligament is markedly stretched and could be pushed dorsally by the advancing endoscope. Diagnosis: severe tracheal collapse. (A ten-year-old Yorkshire terrier with a two-year history of a dry, honking cough induced by excitement.)

46 Tracheal collapse. At the thoracic inlet, the tracheal rings are almost flattened and there is a wide tracheal ligament. Ventrally on the floor of the trachea is a raised, pale area of mucosa with a circular, red, depressed centre, indicative of a contact ulcer (arrow). (A 14-year-old Yorkshire terrier presented in respiratory distress.)

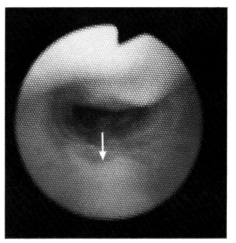

46

Oslerus (Filaroides) osleri infection

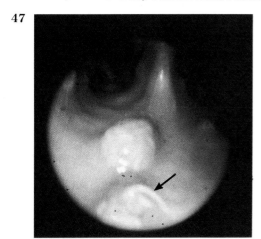

47

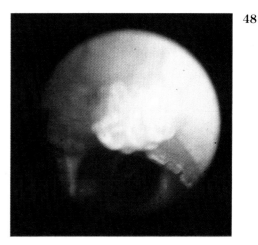

48

47 *O. osleri* infection. There is a large *Filaroides* nodule on the dorsolateral aspect of the trachea, just proximal to the bifurcation. Intertwined adult worms (arrow) are visible. (A one-year-old greyhound imported from Ireland with a chronic cough.)

48 *O. osleri* infection. On the floor of the trachea, proximal to the bifurcation, there are two medium-sized nodules, both filled with adult parasites. The near nodule shows a worm projecting into the lumen of the trachea. In the distance there are a number of smaller nodules in the main bronchi. (A one-year-old Dalmatian with a paroxysmal, exercise-induced, dry cough.)

49 *O. osleri* **infection.** This is a mild infestation showing smaller nodules extending into the second generation bronchi. (A four-year-old yellow Labrador used as a gun dog developed a cough six months prior to presentation.)

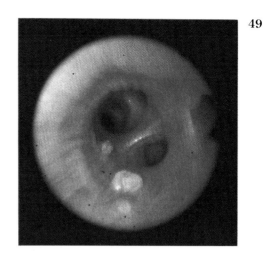

49

50 *O. osleri* **infection.** Following a one-month course of fenbendazole, some small nodules were evident with no worms apparently present. Inflammation and hyperplasia of the mucosa in the second generation bronchi are present, and have caused narrowing of the lumen. (A two-year-old greyhound with *Filaroides* was treated with fenbendazole.)

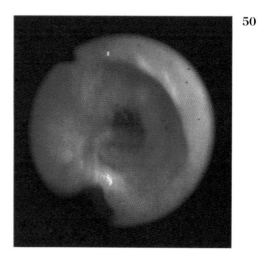

50

51 *O. osleri* **infection.** The same dog as shown in **50** after a further one month's treatment with fenbendazole. No nodules were found, but the mucosa is still friable as the endoscope has induced a small focal haemorrhage on the ventral aspect of the bifurcation of the trachea.

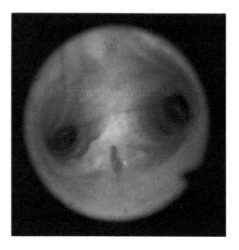

51

Nodular hyperplastic tracheobronchitis

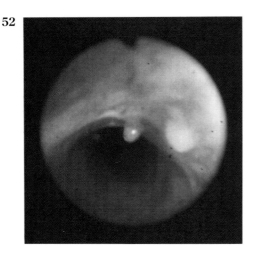

52 Nodular hyperplastic tracheobronchitis. There are two small nodules present in the thoracic trachea. Both nodules are pink-grey and glistening. The mucosa is inflamed in patches and shows some mucosal haemorrhage. Areas of pale mucosa suggestive of scarring are interspersed. (A ten-year-old whippet presented with a six-month history of coughing.)

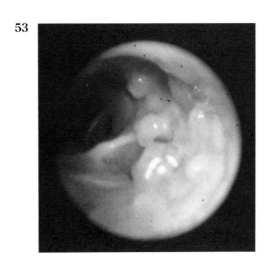

53 Nodular hyperplastic tracheobronchitis in the same dog as in **52**. In the main bronchi there is a large number of these pink-grey nodules of slightly different sizes. There is no evidence of worms in the nodules.

Tracheal foreign body

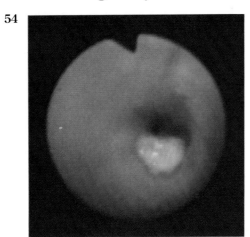

54 Tracheal foreign body. Occupying much of the lumen is a foreign body that was embedded in the mucosa at the bifurcation of the trachea. This was removed with forceps and found to be a piece of a pine cone. (A five-year-old cat with sudden-onset coughing, unresponsive to antibiotics.)

55 Tracheal foreign body. An endotracheal tube with a ragged chewed end can be seen lodged in the trachea. The tracheal mucosa is inflamed and there is mucus mixed with haemorrhage surrounding the narrow tube used for inflating the cuff. (A dog which had a traumatic recovery from anaesthesia, and had only part of the endotracheal tube removed.)

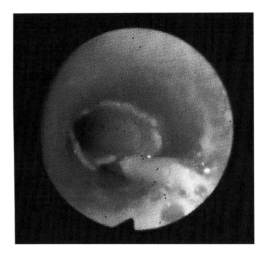

55

Bronchial foreign body

56 Bronchial foreign body. In the right caudal lobe bronchus, a head of wheat is visible, coated in mucopurulent debris. The bifurcation is evident as a pale pillar in the near field. (A springer spaniel with sudden-onset coughing after running in a wheat field.)

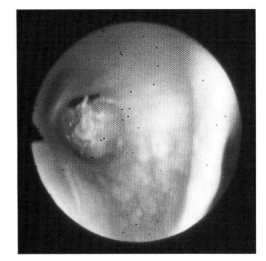

56

57 & 58 Bronchial foreign body. The foreign body, a head of wheat, can be seen projecting from the lumen of a tertiary bronchus. Closer inspection reveals that it is already covered by secretions. The volume of secretion increases rapidly the longer the foreign body is present, and can obscure the foreign body. (A springer spaniel presented with sudden-onset coughing.)

57

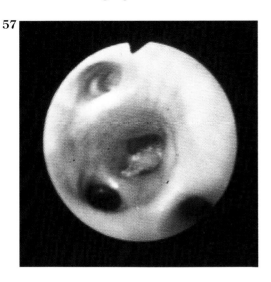

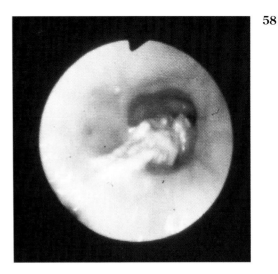

58

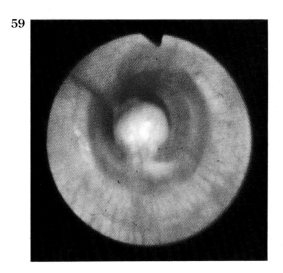

59 Neoplasia. On the floor of the trachea is a discrete, pale, spherical mass. It is attached to the trachea by a broad pedicle. This proved to be a hamartoma. (A three-month-old puppy presented with obstructive dyspnoea.)

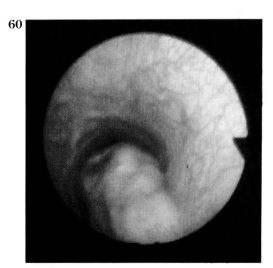

60 Neoplasia. A large, irregular, sessile mass is present on the floor of the trachea. The opposing mucosa is swollen, with an aberrant vascular pattern. This was confirmed histologically as a chondrosarcoma. (A seven-year-old St. Bernard with coughing and inspiratory stridor.)

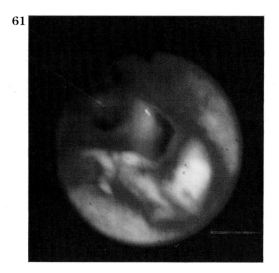

61 Neoplasia. There is fresh blood lying in the lumen of the left main bronchus and some purulent material is emerging from a ventrally located bronchus. The lumen is no longer annular as it is compressed eccentrically by the surrounding tumour mass. (A nine-year-old beagle presented with coughing and haemoptysis.)

5 Upper alimentary tract endoscopy

Introduction

Endoscopic examination of the upper alimentary tract permits examination of the mucosal surface and, to a certain extent, submucosal tissue, without resort to surgical intervention. Apart from the risks of anaesthesia, there have been no recorded complications in the dog or cat as a result of endoscopy of the upper alimentary tract. The radiation hazards that are inevitable with the exposures required for a barium examination, whether by serial films or using image intensifiers, are avoided. Exploratory surgery may still be necessary, but it can follow on from the endoscopic procedure. Surgery may be required if no abnormalities are visible on endoscopy but a lesion is still suspected, or where submucosal tissue is required; most biopsy forceps will barely reach the submucosa.

Endoscopy of the tract is a rapid procedure and one that is easily learned. The pitfalls for the beginner lie in orientation, and recognition of the normal variation in the endoscopic appearance of the stomach in particular.

The principle indication for oesophagoscopy is chronic regurgitation associated with a foreign body, reflux oesophagitis, stricture, and neoplasia (usually benign). Chronic vomiting is associated with several conditions of the stomach and upper duodenum that may be assessed endoscopically: neoplasia, ulceration, hypertrophic gastritis, foreign body and extraluminal lesions.

Choice of instrument

The oesophagus can be examined with either a rigid or a flexible endoscope, but for the stomach and duodenum, flexible instruments are essential. Flexible endoscopes should be panendoscopes, that is, forward viewing (see p.11). In general, panendoscopes are most suited to veterinary work, as they are more versatile than side-viewing instruments and can be used to examine a number of systems. Only those flexible endoscopes which are equipped with facilities for irrigation and insufflation make satisfactory instruments for examining the upper alimentary tract.

Technique

Preparation

Since the stomach should always form part of the examination, except where an oesophageal foreign body is to be removed, the animal should have been starved of food for 18–24 hours and deprived of water for 4–8 hours.

The dog and cat must be anaesthetised to permit adequate examination of the upper gastrointestinal tract. General anaesthesia should be preceded by premedication, avoiding the use of atropine. The specific induction agent is unimportant, but all animals should be intubated to ensure that:

- Fluids which may be present in the oesophagus cannot run forward and enter the trachea.

- Patency of the airway is maintained during manipulation of a foreign body, particularly when a rigid endoscope is used.

Insertion

Care should always be taken to direct the endoscope over the middle of the tongue to avoid the sharp edges of the teeth which may damage the endoscope casing. Passage through the cricopharynx usually causes a 'red-out' as the endoscope abuts on and pushes apart the mucosa. This area is best examined *per os* using a laryngoscope, but it can be adequately visualised when the instrument is withdrawn.

Oesophagoscopy

The caudal thoracic oesophagus is normally dilated when examined, and the cardia can be seen with a variable number of radiating folds or plicae set at an angle to the long axis of the oesophagus. The cardia is normally closed, but when open, the oesophageal mucosa is pale grey-pink and marginates with the red gastric mucosa. This junction is irregular and in man is known as the 'Z-line'.

Gastroscopy

Left lateral recumbency should be used initially, as this allows the pooling of any residual fluid in the fundus. The fundus rarely has lesions that are not present elsewhere. The table should be raised to a height that does not require bending of the junction between the tube and the handpiece of the endoscope, as this avoids extra strain on the control wires. Problems of examination are usually associated with the presence of food, fluid or foam.

A small volume of air is required to separate the walls of the stomach. The part of the gastric mucosa seen initially is the greater curvature of the body. The fold of tissue created by the incisure angularis is an easy landmark to locate, and one that allows orientation for the inexperienced.

Unless the stomach has been overinsufflated, the endoscope can be directed along the lesser curvature into the antrum, where the pylorus may be examined. In many cases, peristaltic waves can be observed and this helps to determine the significance of what may appear to be thickened rugae.

The cardia and fundus can only be properly examined with a panendoscope if the endoscope has been retroflexed. To perform this, the endoscope is either bent around the stomach wall to look back towards the cardia or by using the bending section on those instruments which have a 180° bending capability.

Duodenum

The duodenum cannot be examined in all patients; those that are too large or too small will not allow passage of the endoscope into the duodenum. Lack of success does not automatically indicate a pathological condition.

Oesophagus

Normal endoscopic appearance

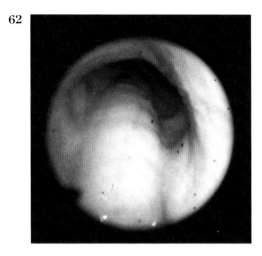

62 **Cervical oesophagus.** In the cervical oesophagus the endotracheal tube and the trachea impinge on the lumen of the oesophagus. Slight insufflation is needed to separate the mucosa as the endoscope is passed distally. This is not needed in the thoracic oesophagus.

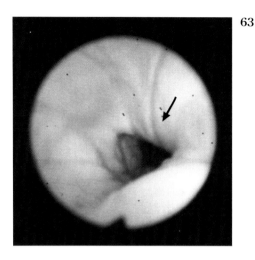

63 **Mid oesophagus.** At the level of the heart base, the aorta (arrow) can usually be seen to impinge on the lumen as the aorta swings dorsally and caudally. The normal longitudinal folds in the mucosa are visible and the margins between the folds appear as dark lines. The mucosa is a pale grey-pink, but in some heavily pigmented dogs, such as the Chow Chow, the mucosa can appear black.

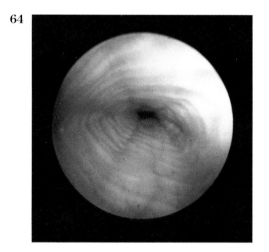

64 **Caudal oesophagus.** Rather than longitudinal folding, annular ridges (the 'herringbone' pattern) are seen in the cat's caudal thoracic oesophagus.

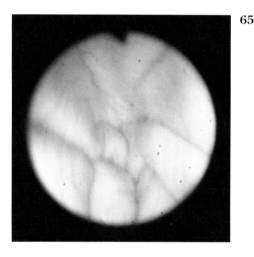

65 **Cardia.** The cardia is normally closed and the longitudinal folds merge to form a series of small radial folds called plicae. The cardia is set at a variable angle to the long axis of the stomach.

Abnormal endoscopic appearance

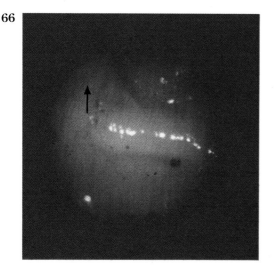

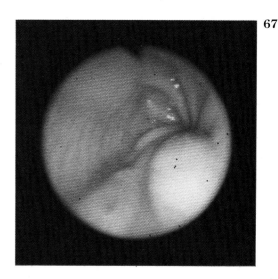

66 Congenital lesions. A large, dilated oesophagus is visible and, at the level of the heart, a thick, extraluminal band of tissue impinges on the oesophagus. Endoscopically, this was seen to originate from a right-sided aorta (arrow). Diagnosis: megaoesophagus secondary to vascular ring anomaly. (An eight-week-old whippet puppy with a four-week history of regurgitation that had increased in severity once solid food had been introduced to its diet.)

67 Congenital lesion. The normal, herringbone mucosal pattern is apparent. However, the normal, fine plicae of the cardia are not visible, and thick rugal folds are present proximal to the hiatus. Hiatus hernia was diagnosed, and confirmed on fluoroscopic examination. (A one-year-old Siamese cat with a history of chronic vomiting that was not always associated with feeding.)

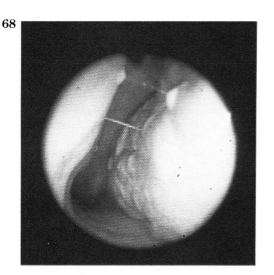

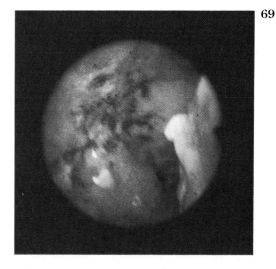

68 Oesophageal obstruction. The oesophageal lumen is occupied by a large, irregular-surfaced mass stretching from the cricopharyngeal area 8–10 cm down the oesophagus. The mass, which caused no resistance to the passage of the endoscope, bears a strong resemblance to a tonsil. (A ten-year-old cairn terrier with episodes of choking, gagging and some respiratory distress. In the pharynx, the right tonsil was missing, but stretching from the tonsillar crypt through the cricopharynx was a thin stalk. This was retracted to deliver a large tonsillar polyp into the oral cavity.)

69 Oesophageal obstruction. Causing an incomplete obstruction, the edge of a bone can be seen. The mucosa is ulcerated, with a very irregular surface covered by fresh blood. (A seven-year-old West Highland white terrier that had been offered a pork chop bone five weeks prior to presentation.)

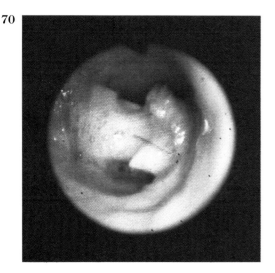

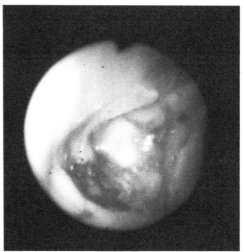

70 Oesophageal obstruction. A bone covered in soft tissue is wedged across the oesophagus, causing about 50% obstruction. There is some swelling and inflammation of the mucosa at the impingement sites.

71 Oesophageal obstruction. Following removal, the damage that has been caused by the projections of the typical, bony, foreign bodies is evident. The mucosa is swollen and ulcerated, with a ragged, bloody, raised lip of mucosa, behind which is a deep defect in the mucosa. Removal often stimulates some bleeding.

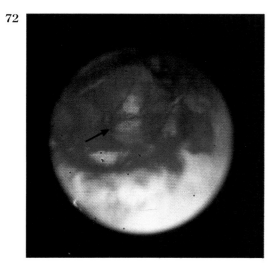

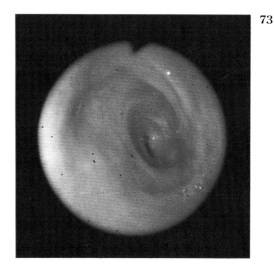

72 Oesophageal obstruction. Appearance of the mucosa following removal of a bone. A swollen rim of mucosa bounds a large, blood-filled crater caused by the bone. In the distance the cardia can be seen (arrow).

73 Stricture. Distal to the heart, the line of the oesophagus is curved rather than straight. The lumen is ovoid and the mucosa is more red than normal. There are a number of thin, white, incomplete, annular ridges projecting into the lumen. All of these abnormalities represent underlying fibrosis, which has created a stricture of some length. The length of the stricture could not be determined as the endoscope could not be passed any further distally, despite the deceptively wide lumen. (A ten-year-old Yorkshire terrier with regurgitation of solid food. The dog had stolen a hot piece of steak from a table, gulping the meat down and running away when discovered.)

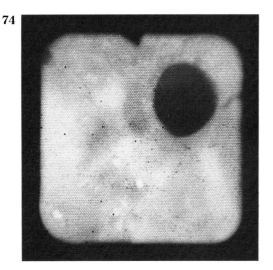

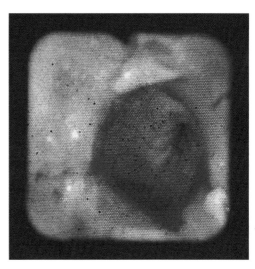

74 & 75   Stricture. There is a narrow stricture that did not allow passage of the endoscope. The mucosa proximal to the stricture is white with several small areas of ulceration. Brushing the endoscope against the mucosa induced haemorrhage. Diagnosis: post-anaesthetic reflux

oesophagitis and stricture. After dilatation with flexible bougies, the lumen has doubled in size and fronds of mucosa are visible. (A two-year-old rough collie following ovariohysterectomy. The dog vomited small amounts of fresh blood mixed with saliva.)

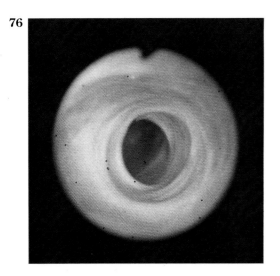

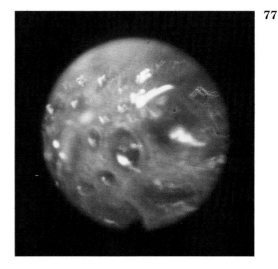

76   Stricture. A series of annular and semiannular fibrous strands can be seen narrowing the lumen of this dog. This was a case of postanaesthetic reflux oesophagitis after one month of intensive anti-stricture chemotherapy including metoclopramide, cimetidine, corticosteroids and antibiotics.

77   Rupture. Following removal and reintroduction of the endoscope, blood-stained fluid is seen bubbling in time with respiration at the site of removal, indicating a rupture of the oesophagus. (A 14-year-old Yorkshire terrier presented with a foreign body that was removed with apparent ease.)

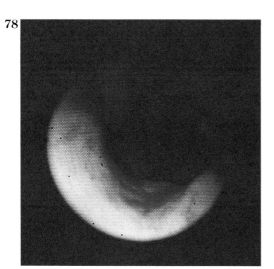

78 Rupture. There is a large, dark hole in the wall of the midcervical portion of the oesophagus. The rim of the defect is smooth, with a small degree of inflammation of the edge. This rupture was successfully repaired. (A six-year-old collie following pharyngeal stick penetration.)

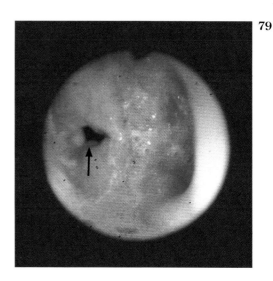

79 Diverticulum. In this eight-month-old cat with a diverticulum the cardia can be seen in the distance as a dark hole (arrow). The mucosal surface of the far wall of the diverticulum is ulcerated, with areas of haemorrhage. The near wall of the diverticulum is in the foreground.

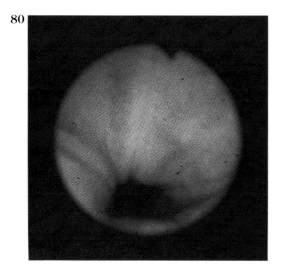

80 Oesophagitis. At the level of the cardia, there are linear erythematous erosions along the centre of the longitudinal folds. (An eight-year-old Labrador with a mast cell tumour admitted for evaluation.)

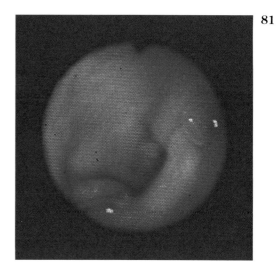

81 Oesophagitis. The mucosa at the cardia is markedly reddened and has exaggerated folding. There is no obvious ulceration, but the abrasion by the endoscope caused mild haemorrhage. The final diagnosis was reflux oesophagitis, but the underlying cause was not identified. (A four-year-old, domestic short-haired cat presented with a one-year history of vomiting and intermittent reluctance to eat.)

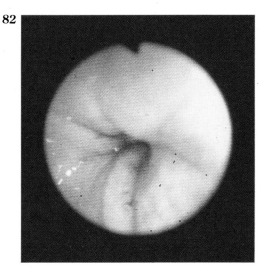

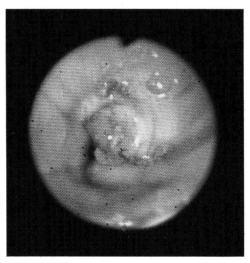

82 Neoplasia. At the cardia, the lower half of the plicae appears normal, albeit a little more stubby than usual. The other half is absent and is replaced by three, large, flat folds that failed to disappear when the cardia was opened. The overlying mucosa is paler than normal. A large ulcer was found on the lesser curvature, typical of gastric carcinoma. These changes were indicative of a retrograde spread of the gastric carcinoma. (A ten-year-old Irish setter with a one-month history of vomiting, weight loss and polydipsia.)

83 Neoplasia. The oesophageal lumen is narrowed by a large, ulcerated mass – an oesophageal sarcoma in a dog imported from Tanzania. *Spirocerca lupi* was implicated.

Stomach

Normal endoscopic appearance

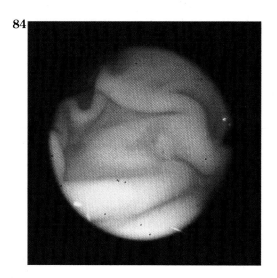

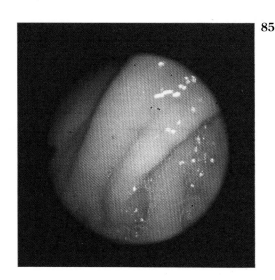

84 Normal rugae. Rugal folding on the greater curvature of the body. This is usually the first area seen on entering the stomach.

85 Normal rugae. A closer view of folds similar to those in **84**. Rugal folds vary in colour from light pink through to red, depending on the angle of reflection of the transmitted light. The bubbled appearance of the small volume of gastric juice present is normal.

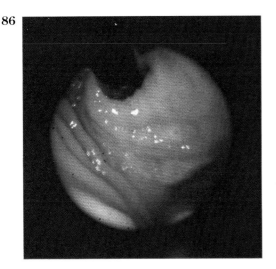

86 Normal cardia. The endoscope has been retroflexed; that is, bent so that it is J-shaped, thus allowing the cardia to be examined. The insertion tube of the endoscope can be seen coming through the cardia. Since the cardia is not gaping, no insufflated air will escape. The fundus is on the left of the picture and the lesser curvature and antrum are in the distance on the right.

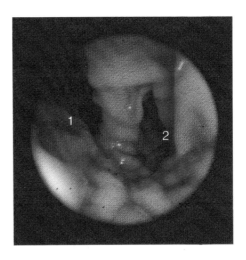

87 Incisure angularis. The endoscope has been passed into the stomach so that the tube is bent around the greater curvature to allow further examination of the incisure angularis. The incisure angularis stands out as a pillar between the fundus (1) and pylorus (2), with rugal folds running across it in the barely inflated stomach.

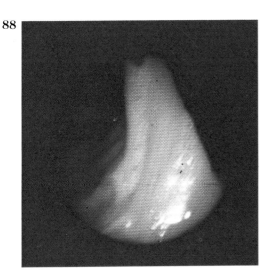

88 Incisure angularis. A closer view of the incisure shown in **87**, once the stomach has been filled with more air. The incisure is again identifiable as a pillar. To the left is the body and the fundus, to the right the antrum.

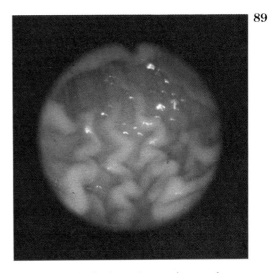

89 Normal body. As the endoscope is passed into the stomach, with as little insufflation as possible, the rugal folds of the greater curvature of the body are visible, normally as tall as they are wide. Dorsally, at the level of the eyepiece marker, is the incisure angularis. Note that when this is viewed from different angles it may have a varied appearance.

90

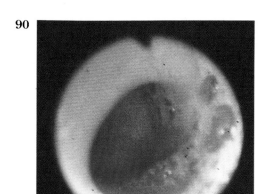

90 Normal antrum. If the endoscope is further advanced into the antrum and canal, the pylorus or pyloric sphincter may be evaluated. As the endoscope advances, it forces the pylorus open and the duodenum can be seen as a smooth-walled tube curving into the distance.

91

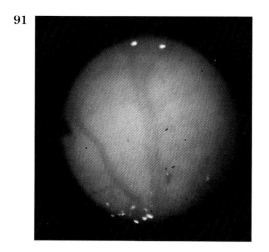

92

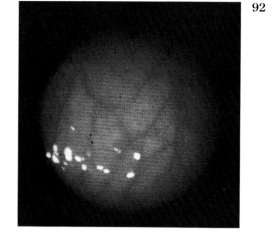

91 & 92 Normal mucosa. When the stomach is well inflated, the submucosal vascular pattern should be visible. Absence of this pattern, where the mucosa appears white, is suggestive of submucosal infiltration.

93

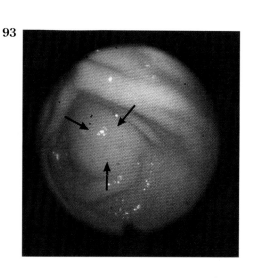

93 Normal artefact. If the stomach is not carefully examined prior to insufflation and the insufflation is then marked, a pseudotumour (arrows) may occasionally be seen. Pseudotumours are usually seen as intraluminal, mural projections in the antrum and pyloric canal on the greater curvature. They are caused by the inflated stomach moulding itself to adjacent organs such as the spleen.

94 Normal artefact. Introduction of the endoscope frequently leads to 'red-out', where the viewing field appears red and no structures are discernible. 'Red-out' occurs because the endoscope abuts on to the wall of the body on the greater curvature. The endoscope should not be forced forwards, but withdrawn, and the stomach gently insufflated. If the end-piece is pushed forwards without such insufflation, it will damage the mucosa, giving rise to a small erosion or bleeding point which may be mistaken by the unwary for a pathological, as opposed to an iatrogenic, lesion.

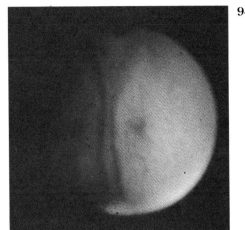

Abnormal endoscopic appearance

95 Congenital pyloric stenosis. The fundus, body and antrum appear normal, but the pyloric sphincter area had a narrow lumen that failed to dilate and permit the passage of the endoscope. (A six-month-old Staffordshire bull terrier with a five-month history of vomiting copious volumes of food and fluid. Latterly, the owner had noticed the abdomen swelling after meals.)

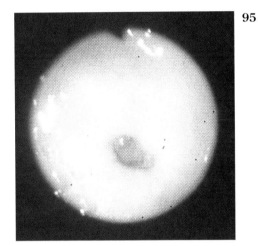

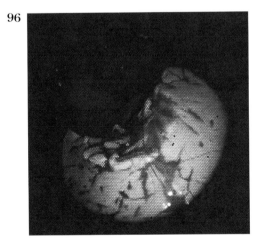

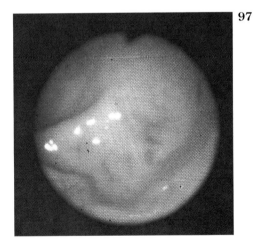

96 & 97 Foreign body. A small piece of wood-effect plastic is visible, and around the fundus and the antrum are areas of inflammation and erosion. (A four-year-old Jack Russell terrier was referred because of frequent vomiting that had proved unresponsive to symptomatic treatment. Plain and contrast radiographs were unremarkable.)

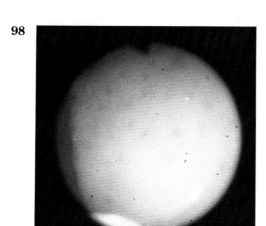

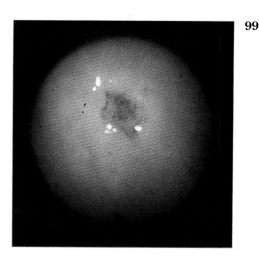

98 Foveolar gastritis. The mucosa is normal in colour, but dotted regularly throughout are red spots, giving an appearance very similar to measles. (A four-year-old Irish setter with a six-month history of intermittent vomiting on an empty stomach.)

99 Erosive gastritis. There is a small erosion approximately 7 mm in diameter. The edge is irregular, with a slightly raised, pale mucosal rim. The base has a number of old bleeding points. (A two-year-old cat with five-day bouts of daily vomiting.)

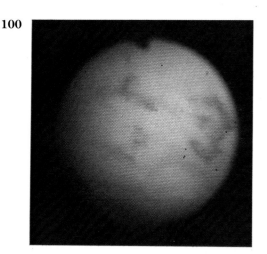

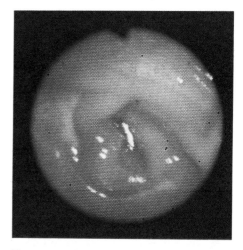

100 Erosive gastritis. A large number of irregular erosions, which in some areas have merged, are visible.

101 Hypertrophic gastritis. Looking up the pyloric canal from the antrum, the mucosa is thrown into large folds that failed to disappear during peristalsis. The surface of some of the hypertrophied folds is inflamed and eroded. (A four-year-old Tibetan spaniel with a one-year history of vomiting. Initially the vomiting had occurred shortly after feeding, but as time elapsed, the gap between feeding and vomiting lengthened, and the vomitus changed in nature from food to fluid. The owner also noticed that the dog's abdomen tended to swell after eating, and that this ballooning abated once the animal had vomited.)

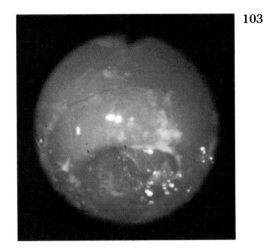

102 Hypertrophic gastritis. A normal, wide antrum is not visible from the body looking towards the antrum, but the lumen is narrowed by thick hypertrophied and inflamed rugal folds.

103 Duodenogastric reflux. The orange tinge to the mucus is due to the bile reflux, beneath which the mucosa is inflamed. (A four-year-old springer spaniel with a three-month history of daily vomiting. The owners were often awakened in the early hours of the morning by the dog's vomiting, or would find a small puddle of bile-stained vomit on the floor.)

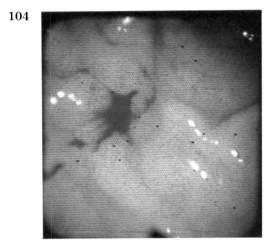

104 Peptic ulcer. Five rugal folds of normal thickness and height can be seen running into a small area that is slightly raised from the surrounding mucosa at the junction of the body and the antrum. Fresh blood masks the ulcer base. (A two-year-old German shepherd dog with a six-month history of haematemesis and dark, tarry stools.)

105 Peptic ulcer. A small (1 cm diameter) ulcer is visible at the junction of the incisure angularis and the dorsal wall. The flat base is filled with a small amount of debris and some blood. The rim barely rises above the surrounding normal mucosal surface. (A five-year-old West Highland white terrier had a one-year history of vomiting on an empty stomach. The vomitus was generally white, but often had a 'coffee ground' appearance. The signs tended to occur in bouts accompanied by abdominal pain, with intervening periods of normality.)

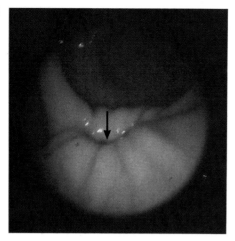

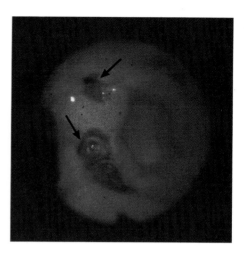

106   Peptic ulcer. A discrete (1.5 cm diameter) ulcer (arrow) is found at the base of the visceral or dorsal end of the pillar created by the incisure angularis. The ulcer is barely elevated from the surrounding mucosa, and a number of normal rugal folds can be seen running into the rim, which is quite smooth and regular in outline. The antrum can be seen in the distance as a dark shadow. (A two-year-old Dobermann pinscher presented with sudden onset profuse haematemesis of four days' duration.)

107   Peptic ulcer. Two ulcers (arrows) are visible on the incisure angularis. Both have dark bases filled with blood. To the right is the antrum. (A six-year-old Jack Russell terrier with sudden onset haematemesis, four days after initiation of non-steroidal anti-inflammatory therapy. The maturity of the ulcers suggested that they were pre-existing and that the non-steroidal drugs precipitated the massive bleeding.)

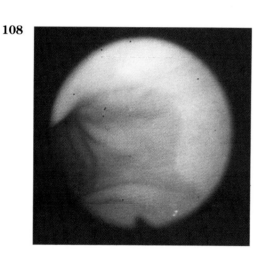

108   Gastric carcinoma. The oesophagogastric junction is gaping and the 'Z-line' is visible. This is abnormal and usually associated with the submucosal retrograde spread of a tumour, in this case a gastric carcinoma. (A ten-year-old Irish setter with a one-month history of frequent vomiting.)

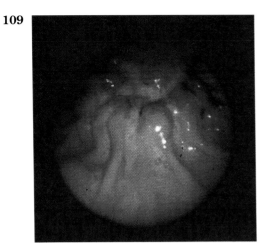

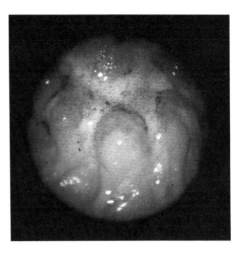

109 & 110   Gastric carcinoma. A large (6 cm diameter) markedly elevated ulcer is present on the lesser curvature. A large number of rugal folds can be seen running up the outer wall and broadening out as they merge with the rim. The rim is irregular and the inner wall is ulcerated. (A nine- year-old Shetland collie had a two-month history of vomiting, occasionally producing brown vomitus. The dog had lost a considerable amount of weight, although this was not apparent to the owner because of the coat, showed a marked increase in thirst and passed very dark stools.)

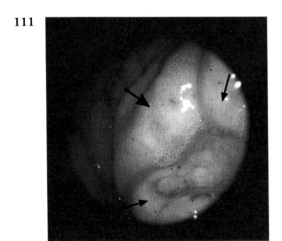

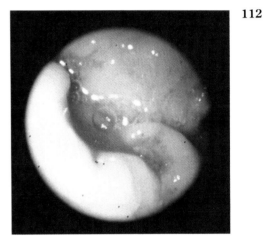

111   Gastric carcinoma. In this skyline view of a large ulcer (large arrow) at the incisure, which was no longer identifiable, a very thick rim (small arrows) to the ulcer can be seen, with some areas of superficial ulceration. An excavated inner wall with an overhanging rim is visible.

112   Gastric carcinoma. A large (5 cm diameter) mass is present on the lesser curvature of the body of the stomach, with the ulcer rising above the surrounding mucosa. The outer wall is pale and the rim is thick and ragged. (A 12-year-old, domestic short-haired cat with a two-month history of repeated vomiting episodes.)

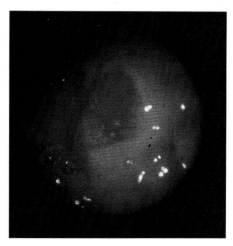

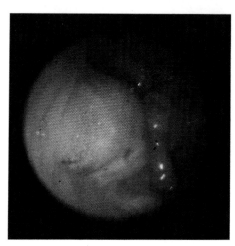

113 Gastric lymphosarcoma. An ulcer is present, the base of which is shallow relative to the rim. Numerous other marginally raised ulcers, 2–3 cm in diameter, were seen throughout the stomach, most having evidence of active or recent bleeding. (A four-year-old German shepherd dog was seen to be losing weight, and was reluctant to eat and exercise. Daily examination of the kennel revealed puddles of brown vomitus with patches of unchanged blood.)

114 Gastric lymphosarcoma. This large ulcer of the fundus is raised above the surrounding mucosa, and the rim is much wider than is usually seen with gastric carcinoma. Focal areas of inflamed and superficially ulcerated mucosa surround the protuberant ulcer. (A three-year-old German shepherd dog with a six-month history of recurrent vomiting and abdominal pain, unassociated with food.)

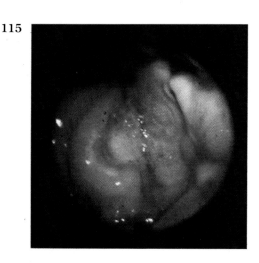

115 Gastric lymphosarcoma. The large, malignant ulcer at the incisure angularis has a thick, irregular rim and an ulcerated inner wall. It is indistinguishable endoscopically from gastric carcinoma. (A six-year-old, domestic long-haired cat was a known scavenger and its frequent vomiting was put down to its nightly forays. However, the persistent nature of the vomiting, polydipsia and weight loss made the owner seek veterinary attention).

6 Lower alimentary tract endoscopy

Introduction

Endoscopy of the lower gastrointestinal tract is indicated in patients with signs of tenesmus, dyschezia, haematochezia, constipation, or chronic 'large bowel' diarrhoea (characterised by frequent passage of small volumes of faeces with fresh blood and/or mucus). Visual examination of lesions at endoscopy, together with microscopic examination of mucosal biopsies, can be used to discriminate between the various types of colitis, colonic tumours and caecal inversion. Endoscopic examination is more likely to yield a definitive diagnosis than specialised radiographic studies, which to a large extent have been rendered obsolete by the increased availability of endoscopic equipment. However, gastrointestinal tumours can be submucosal, and endoscopy will be unrewarding and endoscopic biopsies unrepresentative.

Faecal examination and cytological examination of rectal mucosal scrapings may reveal evidence of endemic parasites (*Ancylostoma*, *Trichuris*), or other infections (*Histoplasma capsulatum*). Treatment with fenbendazole for potential occult whipworm infection is often warranted before a complete endoscopic examination.

Choice of instrument

The descending colon and rectum can be examined with a rigid endoscope (**116**), but a fibreoptic endoscope or videoendoscope (**117**) is needed to evaluate the transverse and ascending colon, caecum, ileocolic valve and ileum. Since many colonic diseases involve the mucosa diffusely, rigid colonoscopy is often both economical and effective. However, if available, flexible endoscopy is preferable since the entire large bowel, and often the ileum, can be evaluated.

Technique

Preparation

Complete evacuation of all faeces from the colon prior to endoscopic examination is desirable, although this ideal situation is difficult to achieve consistently. Food must be withheld for at least 36 hours, and preferably for 48–72 hours. For rigid colonoscopic examination, two warm-water enemas (10–20 ml/kg) administered the day before the procedure, and a final enema on the morning of the examination, will usually provide cleansing. Administration of a laxative such as bisacodyl (5 mg for cats, 5–25 mg for dogs) may also aid colonic evacuation, while oral magnesium citrate or sulphate will further increase the effectiveness of these methods.

Colon electrolyte lavage solutions, such as Golytely® (Braintree Laboratories, USA; Seward, UK) or Colyte® (Reed and Carnrick, USA), are preferable for complete bowel cleansing prior to examination of the entire colon with a flexible endoscope. These solutions are not absorbed when administered orally, and, since they contain electrolytes, they do not cause systemic electrolyte or acid-base changes. They are administered via a stomach tube at a dose of 40 ml/kg, given twice (at an interval of 2–4 hours) the day before the procedure, with a repeat dose in the morning of the examination. Metoclopramide (0.3–0.5 mg/kg) may be given with the last dose to facilitate emptying of the stomach prior to anaesthesia. An additional high warm-water enema 1–2 hours before examination will maximise cleansing of the entire large bowel. Unless the effluent is clear, the cleansing will not have been adequate.

Insertion

It is preferable that all patients are anaesthetised, as this reduces discomfort and risk to the patient and damage to the endoscope. Positioning will depend on whether a rigid or a flexible endoscope is being used.

The tip of the lubricated endoscope should be inserted and passed cranially with gentle pressure. Insufflation must be used to allow safe passage of the endoscope, and examination of the mucosa as the instrument is advanced, thus minimising the risk of perforation. It also allows the recognition of artefactual lesions of the colonic lining, and in particular, small areas of haemorrhage, and linear mucosal reddening in the rectum which may reflect trauma secondary to administration of enemas and should not be over-interpreted.

Since many flexible endoscopes are relatively narrow in diameter, air tends to escape through the anal sphincter, and it may help if an assistant applies pressure manually to the anus in order to prevent egress of air. Rotation and redirection are frequently required to traverse the splenic and hepatic flexures, and at these positions a clear view of the lumen may be impossible for a few centimetres.

If masses are identified, repeated biopsy samples from the same site are often useful, since superficial tissue may reveal only nonspecific inflammatory change, while evidence of neoplasia may be found in deeper tissue. Cytological as well as histological examination may more reliably demonstrate the presence of neoplastic cells, and will be particularly helpful in demonstrating agents such as *Histoplasma* or *Prototheca*.

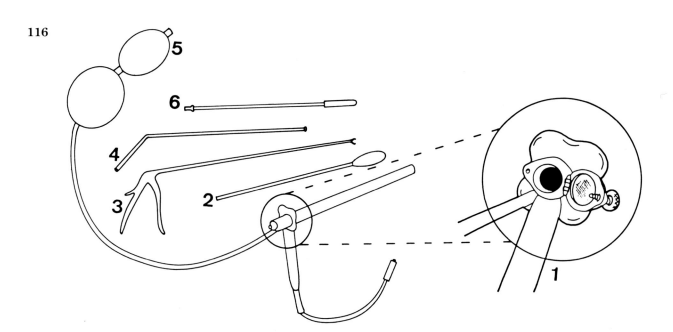

116 Components of a rigid colonoscopy system. The obturator (6) is placed in the lumen of the endoscope only to facilitate passage through the anus. The light source is located in the handle of the endoscope near to the eyepiece (1). The viewing lens is closed over the eyepiece to magnify the image and retain air in the colon during insufflation by means of a hand-operated pump (5). Residual faecal matter may be removed by the use of large cotton-tipped swabs (2) or by suction applied to a smooth-ended tube (4) passed down the lumen of the endoscope. Cutting biopsy forceps (3) are passed down the lumen of the endoscope to obtain samples of colonic mucosa.

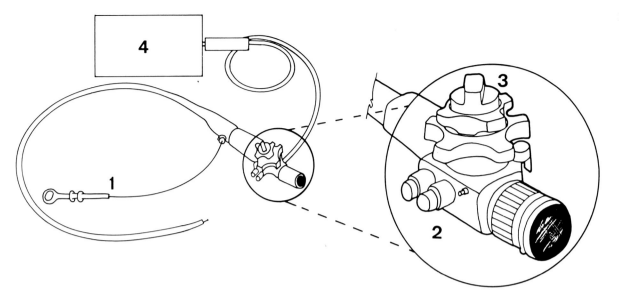

117   Components of a flexible endoscopic system suitable for examination of the lower gastro-intestinal tract. The light source (4) is a separate unit and light is passed to the tip of the endoscope through fibreoptic bundles. After insertion of the endoscope both suction and delivery of air or water to the tip of the instrument are regulated by buttons on its handle (2). The tip is directed by means of wires attached to control knobs (3). Flexible forceps (1) may be passed down a dedicated channel in the endoscope.

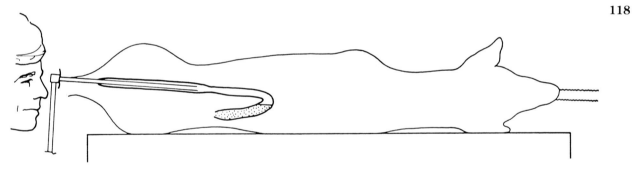

118   Positioning the patient for rigid colonoscopy. When the patient is in right lateral recumbency the endoscope can be angled so that any residual material drains away from the operator back into the more proximal segments, enhancing mucosal visualisation.

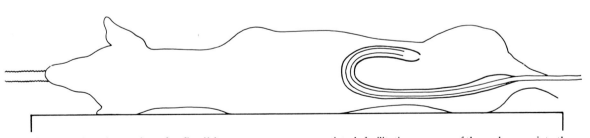

119   Positioning the patient for flexible colonoscopy. When the patient is in left lateral recumbency the splenic and hepatic flexures are more easily negotiated, facilitating passage of the endoscope into the transverse and ascending colon.

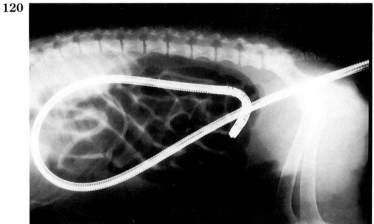

120

121

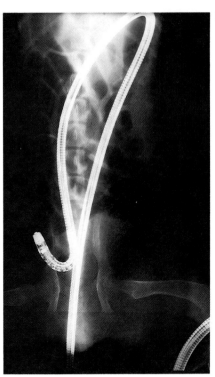

120 & 121   Lateral (120) and ventrodorsal (121) radiographic views of a flexible videoendoscope positioned in the terminal ileum of a dog. Once the ileocolic junction and the adjacent caecal orifice have been identified, the colonoscope will be pointing towards the operator. The small intestine is distended with air following insufflation of the colon to allow passage of the endoscope.

122

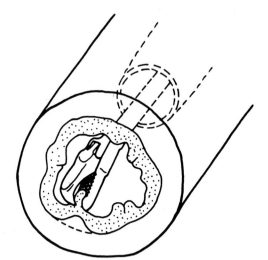

123

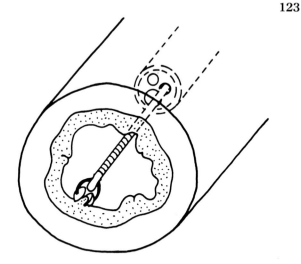

122 & 123   Obtaining mucosal biopsies during rigid (122) and flexible (123) colonoscopy. To minimise the risk of perforation, particular care must be taken to tent the mucosa when using large cutting forceps introduced through a rigid endoscope. The small nips of tissue grasped by flexible endoscopic forceps present little risk of perforation.

Normal endoscopic appearance

124–127 Normal colon. Insufflation of air progressively smooths mucosal folds and allows the endoscope to be advanced with a clear view of the lumen. Failure to distend a segment of the colon or ileum is abnormal, and such stenotic lesions usually reflect neoplastic infiltration or fibrosis secondary to severe inflammation.

128 Normal colon. On insertion of the endoscope, residual faecal matter can often be removed by suction or by swabbing with large, cotton-tipped swabs. Traces of adherent faeces such as those illustrated do not interfere with a complete colonic examination.

129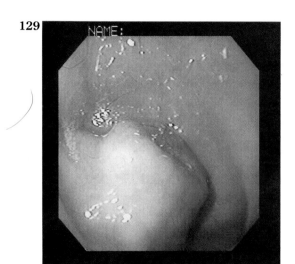

130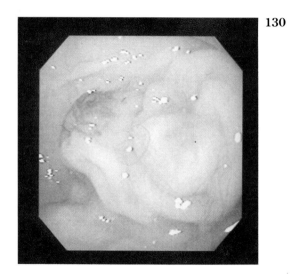

131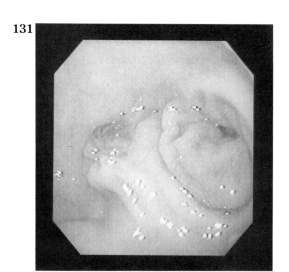

132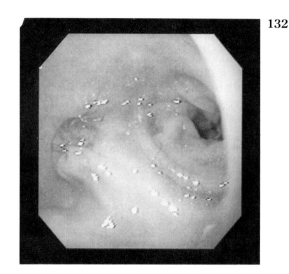

133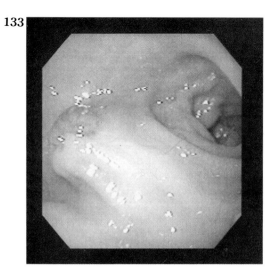

129–133 **Normal ileocolic junction.** The ileocolic junction is usually seen as a closed sphincter on the tip of a mushroom-like protruberance in the lumen of the colon (**129**). The tip of the scope can sometimes be coaxed into the ileum by the application of gentle pressure and alternate insufflation and aspiration of air, together with lubrication by flushing the tip of the scope with water. If this approach is not successful then a biopsy forceps may be passed into the ileum and subsequently used either to obtain biopsies or as a guide wire to facilitate insertion of the scope itself into the lumen. In contrast, the caecocolic junction is frequently open and the lumen of the caecum readily examined. In this series of photographs (**130–133**) the caecal orifice was initially closed (**130**), but the sphincter spontaneously relaxed to produce a more typical appearance (**133**).

134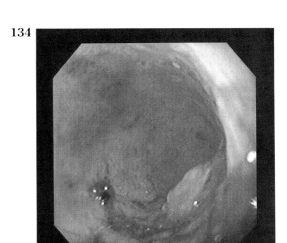

135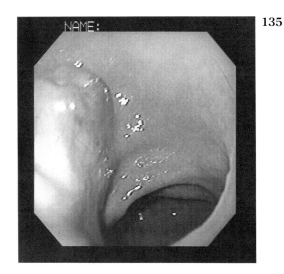

134 & 135 Normal caecum. The caecum of cats is a short, comma-shaped sac (**134**) in contrast to the much longer spiral-shaped organ of the dog (**135**).

136 Normal ileum. Once the ileum has been entered, submucosal blood vessels are not apparent in normal animals. Furthermore, the presence of villi, with dome-shaped tips lining the ileum, leads to multiple, small, reflected images of the endoscope light, giving a velvety appearance to the mucosa, and contrasting sharply with that of normal colonic mucosa.

136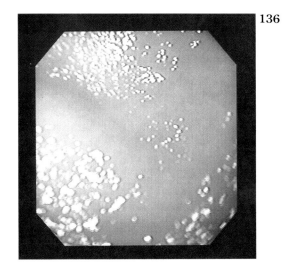

137 Normal colon. The normal colonic mucosa reflects light evenly, and submucosal blood vessels can be readily identified. Disappearance of these vessels is the first sign of oedema or inflammation, and this, coupled with excessive amounts of mucus in the lumen, is the most common abnormal finding in cats and dogs with large bowel disease.

137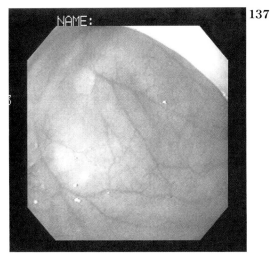

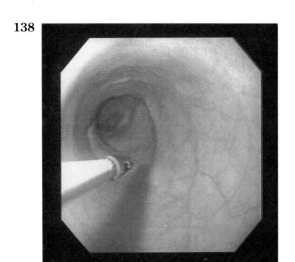
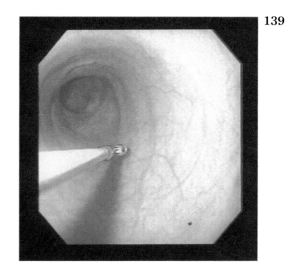

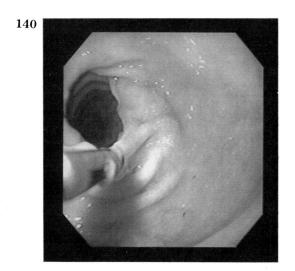
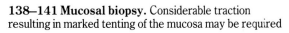
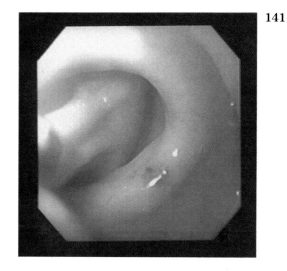

138–141 Mucosal biopsy. Considerable traction resulting in marked tenting of the mucosa may be required to free mucosal biopsies taken with small flexible endoscopic biopsy forceps.

142 Colonic biopsy. There is usually minimal bleeding following biopsy of colonic mucosa, and significant seepage is a sign of mucosal abnormality. Two biopsy sites near the ileocolic sphincter are visible. Tissue had been removed from the site further away from the sphincter two minutes before the picture was taken. The other site was biopsied 30 seconds before the site was photographed. The mucosa was normal on both gross and histological examination.

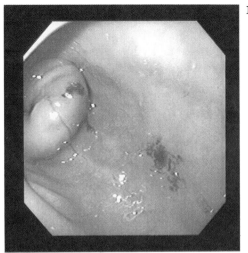

Abnormal endoscopic appearance

Infection

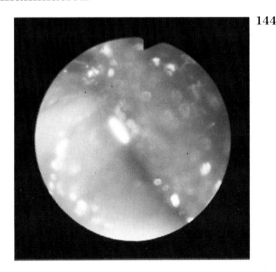

143

143 Histoplasmosis. Colonoscopy revealed numerous haemorrhagic foci, and a friable mucosa that bled excessively after biopsies were taken. Similar, although less dramatic abnormalities were seen in the duodenum. (An eight-year-old, female mixed-breed dog with progressive anorexia, weight loss and watery diarrhoea with occasional flecks of fresh blood and mucus. Biopsies of small and large intestine revealed lymphocytic-plasmacytic infiltration, and cytological examination of touch preparations of the fresh biopsies demonstrated *Histoplasma capsulatum* organisms in association with macrophages. The dog recovered completely following treatment with amphotericin B and ketoconazole.)

Inflammation

144

144 Ileocolic intussusception. The endoscope was easily advanced alongside the prolapsed bowel, demonstrating that the lesion was not caused by rectal prolapse. The hyperaemic mucosa on the right side of the field is ileal, while the paler mucosa on the left side is colonic. The ileal mucosa is distinguished by the granular surface coated with numerous small villus tips that reflect the light from the endoscope. (A three-year-old female greyhound presented with prolapse of a segment of bowel through the anus.)

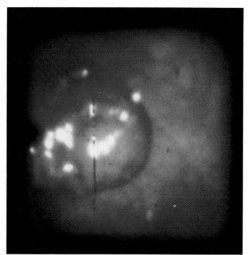

145 Inverted caecum. On colonoscopic examination the tip of an inverted caecum was seen in the lumen of the ascending colon at the hepatic flexure. When the tip of the endoscope was advanced, the totally inverted caecum could be seen emerging from the ileocolic junction. (A three-year-old, female, mixed-breed dog was presented with a three-month history of intermittent but frequent passage of small amounts of faeces. This had been a daily occurrence for two weeks prior to presentation. Surgical resection of the inverted caecum and terminal ileum was followed by resolution of clinical signs.) (Courtesy of Dr Ray Dillon).

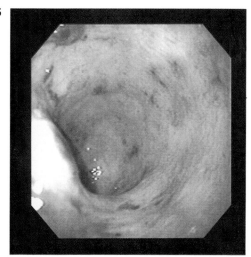

146 Lymphocytic–plasmacytic colitis. Colonoscopic examination revealed a granular appearance to the mucosa, with poor visualization of submucosal blood vessels. There were several small mucosal haemorrhagic areas. After biopsies were taken, the mucosa bled more than is usual. (A four-year-old castrated, male, domestic short-haired cat was presented with several months' history of intermittent diarrhoea characterised by the passage of semiformed stools with mucus and fresh blood. The cat responded favourably to treatment with oral prednisolone.)

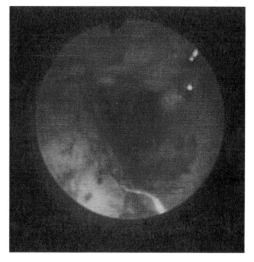

147 Eosinophilic colitis. Colonoscopic examination demonstrated numerous, pinpoint haemorrhagic areas and a granular appearance to the mucosa, with inability to visualise submucosal blood vessels. There was excessive bleeding after mucosal biopsies were taken. (An eleven-year-old, male poodle was presented because of tenesmus, haematochezia, anorexia and weight loss. Therapy with sulphasalazine was followed by the resolution of all clinical signs. A subsequent recurrence of signs responded equally rapidly to administration of oral prednisolone.)

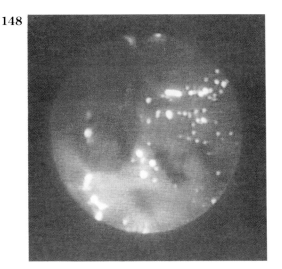

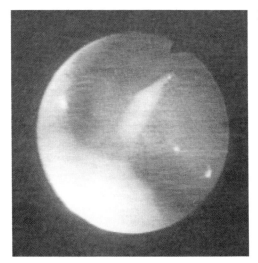

148   Suppurative colitis. At colonoscopy the most dramatic findings were marked hyperaemia of the ileocolic sphincter and patchy haemorrhagic areas of colonic mucosa. (An eight-year-old Rhodesian ridgeback presented with acute onset of severe pain when defaecating. Small amounts of faeces were passed with traces of fresh blood and mucus. The dog showed signs of pain during abdominal palpation and a faecal examination for parasites was negative. Cytological examination of a touch preparation of faeces showed numerous neutrophils. No cause was evident. The dog was treated with fenbendazole (for possible occult parasitism) and sulphasalazine was

administered for four weeks. Clinical signs resolved rapidly and did not recur.)

149   Lymphocytic-plasmacytic enteritis. The submucosal blood vessels were not visible at colonoscopy and a tapeworm segment could be seen. (A seven-year-old cat was presented with chronic diarrhoea characterised by the passage of semiformed faeces with mucus and fresh blood. Biopsy revealed a lymphocytic-plasmacytic infiltrate. Similar histological changes were evident in biopsies taken from the stomach and duodenum. The tapeworm segments were probably an incidental finding.)

Neoplasia

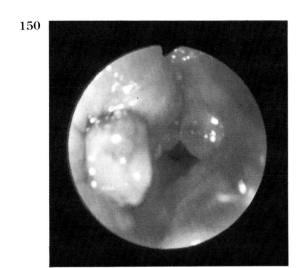

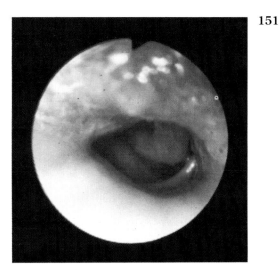

150   Benign polyp. Multiple, ovoid, smooth-surfaced polyps are visible stretching into the distance in the rectal canal. (A two-year-old dog was presented because of tenesmus and haematochezia. The remainder of the large bowel was normal in appearance. The polyps were surgically excised after everting the mucosa through the anus. All clinical signs then resolved.)

151   Rectal lymphosarcoma. The mass is visible as a proliferative intraluminal lesion with a haemorrhagic surface. (A cat was presented with constipation and intermittent haematochezia.) (Courtesy of Dr Colin Burrows).

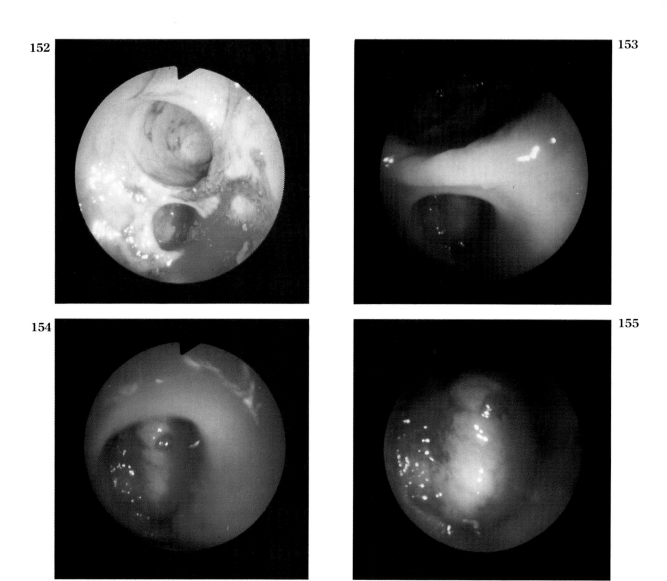

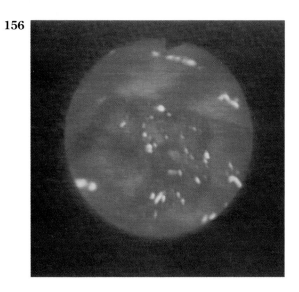

152–155 Leiomyosarcoma. The colon was initially normal on flexible endoscopic examination, but fresh blood was visible passing into the colon from the ileum (**152**). The larger of the two orifices is the entrance to the caecum. As the ileocolic sphincter was approached, it relaxed further (**153**) and a mass became visible (**154**) in the terminal ileum. The mass (**155**) was friable and bled excessively following biopsy. (An eleven-year-old, male German shepherd dog was presented with a history of recurrent episodes of severe acute haematochezia over an eight- month period. Radiological examination was unremarkable. The tumour was completely excised at exploratory laparotomy and there were no subsequent episodes of haematochezia.)

156 Colonic adenocarcinoma. An extremely friable haemorrhagic mass was found almost completely obscuring the colonic lumen, approximately 15 cm from the anus. (A 12-year-old, mixed-breed dog was presented for investigation of severe tenesmus and haematochezia.)

7 Vaginoscopy

Introduction

Vaginoscopy is a relatively simple technique, requiring a modest outlay in terms of equipment. The ease with which repeated examinations can be performed is of particular value when assessing the cyclic bitch.

Vaginoscopy has several indications:

- Suspected congenital or acquired abnormalities.

- In breeding programmes and for investigations of infertility.

- Obstetrical evaluation in abnormal parturition.

- Secondary procedures such as biopsy, foreign-body retrieval, precise smear collection, artificial insemination, transcervical cannulation and post-partum intra-uterine therapy.

Choice of instrument

A rigid endoscope 30 cm long and 4.7 mm in diameter, or a flexible instrument of similar dimensions, allows the length of the vagina and the narrow cranial region to be examined. Endoscopes of greater diameter are limited to larger bitches, and do not permit satisfactory viewing of the cranial vagina or the cervix.

Technique

Patient preparation

Most bitches may be examined in a standing position without chemical restraint, or, at most, under mild sedation. However, for some procedures, general anaesthesia may be required. In heavily coated bitches the perivulval hair should be trimmed or held aside with hair clips. A tail wrap can be used for long, feathered tails. The perineum should be cleaned with a suitable antiseptic solution.

Vaginoscopy is tolerated well by the unsedated, periparturient bitch during all stages of labour and in the early postpartum period, if the pups are contented and within her view. However, in order to facilitate viewing, it may be necessary to remove blood clots or debris either by wiping out the vagina with long, bacteriological swabs or by irrigating it with warm, sterile saline.

Insertion

The assembled endoscope, with its sheath, is introduced in a dorsocranial direction through the vulva into the vestibule up to the ischial arch and then re-angled for the more horizontal vagina. The dorso-cranial insertion minimises trauma. It also avoids striking the clitoral fold and the ischial arch, and inadvertent entry into the urethral meatus. The latter is a problem in obese bitches, where a fat-laden fold may overhang the urethral opening. With a flexible endoscope, the bending section is locked until the vagina is reached, or a short plastic tube may be used as a speculum. In small bitches the cranial vaginal dimensions may be critical and the 4.7 mm rigid endoscope can be inserted without its sheath, through a plastic tube.

Vaginal insufflation is provided by an automatic

insufflator or by a large syringe attached to an endoscope inlet port. Insufflation should be used from the start of an examination for diagnostic purposes, to give a panoramic view. Caution should be exercised when vaginal tears or erosions are suspected. When assessing cyclic status, minimal insufflation is advised in order to avoid mucosal distortion.

All manipulations of the endoscope within the vagina should be made slowly and while viewing, to avoid trauma to the vaginal wall. During cyclic examinations, when the enlarged mucosal folds may obscure vision, partial withdrawal and readvancement of the endoscope may be required. In large bitches, or those with a pendulous abdomen, upward pressure on the abdomen may help to straighten the tract. The mucosa should also be inspected as the endoscope is slowly withdrawn, when many features are more readily observed.

Two areas of resistance are normally encountered during the passage of the endoscope:

- The caudal vaginal sphincter of the vestibulovaginal junction is met first. In a normal, intact bitch only a slight to moderate increase in pressure is required here, but resistance is greater where the tract is quiescent. No force should be used and if much resentment is shown, or strong resistance encountered, the problem should be visually identified while insufflating the vestibule. A psychophysiological, vestibulovaginal stenosis ascribed to 'temperamental' cyclic bitches can respond to mild sedation.

- The second area of resistance is met more cranially, at the caudal tubercle. To view the cervix, insufflation is used to expose the caudal tubercle and the paracervical lumen. Controlled increase in pressure is usually required to advance the endoscope under the caudal tubercle. In many bitches the endoscopist is aware of a distinct, and sometimes quite disconcerting, 'popping' sensation as the endoscope enters the paracervical lumen.

Orientation

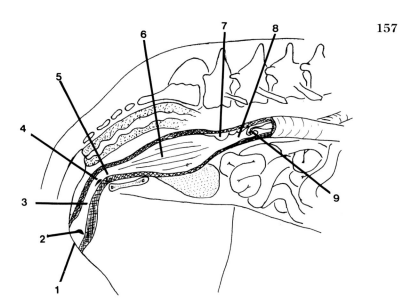

157   Postuterine or caudal reproductive tract of the bitch. Vulva (1), Clitoral fossa (2), Vestibule (3), Urethral meatus (4), Vestibulovaginal junction (5), Caudal vagina (6), Caudal tubercle of dorsal median fold (7), Paracervix (8) and Cervix (9).

There is an almost vertical incline to the vault of the vestibule below the anus, after which it bends sharply to become the more horizontal vagina (**157**). The vestibulovaginal junction forms the base of a bottle-shaped vagina: a large caudal region with primary longitudinal mucosal folds (the body); a short midvaginal region with flatter mucosa (the shoulders); and a much narrower paracervix cranially (the neck of the bottle), with the cervix projecting like a cork from the dorso-cranial extremity.

The paracervix has a crescent-shaped lumen and a longitudinal dorsal median fold which forms a bulbous caudal tubercle where it joins the midvaginal mucosa. At certain stages of the oestrous cycle, middle and cranial tubercles develop between the caudal tubercle and the cervix.

The bulbous cervix is concealed from view by the tubercles of the dorsal median fold. Its apex may touch the paracervical floor, and the external os is directed ventrally. Apical furrows converge towards the recessed, centrally placed os, giving the bulbous cervix a typical squashed 'cash purse' appearance that distinguishes it from the unfurrowed tubercles. The location and mobility of the cervix, together with the upward inclination of its canal, make transcervical cannulation difficult in the bitch. Although the histological junction between endometrial and vaginal mucosae is sharp, the gross junction is irregular, and cervical biopsies may show only some endometrial tissue; similarly, observable changes in the cervix may also be patchy.

Vaginoscopic cyclic changes

A major role for vaginoscopy is the assessment of oestrous status. Hormonally dictated changes imposed on the basic mucosal pattern are sufficiently consistent to determine cyclic status. In particular, the changing profiles of the caudal tubercle, the contours of mucosal folds and summits, mucosal density and colour, and the character and colour of any fluids present are very sensitive indicators. There are four successive periods within an oestrous cycle, differentiated by unique vaginoscopic features:

1 An **oedematous proliferative period**, typified by a mucosal oedema enlarging the primary folds into smooth-walled 'balloons', starts the cycle. Uterine fluid is clear and bright red. The oedematous period coincides with the preovulatory period from cycle-onset to the start of the lutenising hormone (LH) surge, that is, early and mid pro-oestrus.

2 The **non-angulated shrinkage period** is the first of two consecutive phases of progressive mucosal shrinkage that are characterised by the formation of many additional surface furrows and 'secondary' folds, leading to an increase in mucosal pallor and density. In the non-angulated shrinkage period, mucosal summit profiles remain rounded and even, and the uterine fluid tends to become scant and serum-like towards the end of the phase. This stage spans the periovulatory period from the time of the LH surge up to three days post LH peak, when ovulation is most likely, that is, late pro-oestrus.

3 In the succeeding period of **angulated shrinkage**, increasing numbers of mucosal summit profiles become sharply angulated and irregular; the mucosa becomes a dense-cream to paper-white. The uterine fluid remains serum-like. During this period, the oocytes can be fertilised (from about four days post LH peak); behavioural receptivity (that is, standing oestrus) and the time of the 'oestrous smear' coincide in part with the fertilisation period. The optimum time for insemination occurs during this period when angulation is maximal.

4 A period of **decline and cessation of shrinkage**, during which the much 'deflated' mucosa thins and the sharp profiles become more rounded, ends the cycle, and marks the transition to the onset of metoestrus. The vaginal mucus tends to be thick and forms brown, jelly-like ribbons. The decline and cessation of the shrinkage period also marks the end of the fertilisation period; that is, late oestrus into early metoestrus.

In metoestrus the mucosa has simple, longitudinal folds with patchy, pink-white, banded mucosa. When touched with the endoscope, the mucosa tends to pucker into rosettes. Metoestral mucus is abundant, thick and opalescent. During the quiescent phase of anoestrus, the mucosa is thin, diffusely pink, and has a simple, flaccid fold-pattern. Mucus is scant and transparent.

Normal vaginoscopic appearance

158

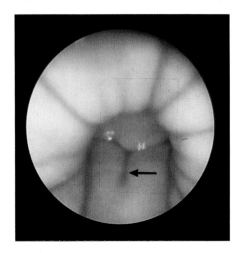

158 Urethral meatus. The slit-like urethral meatus (arrow) lies on the cranioventral floor of the vestibule, proximal to the clitoral fossa and distal to the vestibulo-vaginal junction.

159

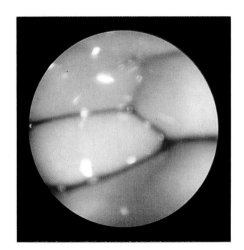

159 Vagina – oedematous proliferative period (early pro-oestrus). The primary folds of the midvagina are seen as large, oedematous balloons of pale pink mucosa. They have a smooth, unwrinkled surface during this phase. Clear red fluid can be seen among the folds.

160

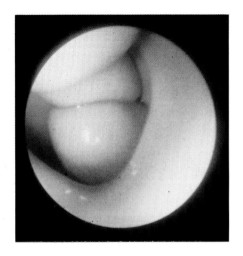

160 Paracervix – oedematous proliferative period (early pro-oestrus). The endoscope tip is under the caudal tubercle (top left). The paracervix has a crescentic shape, and within it can be seen the middle and the cranial tubercles. Note their smooth, unwrinkled and bulbous profiles. The cervix is hidden from view.

161 Cervix – pro-oestrus. The cervix has been displaced by the tip of the endoscope to reveal the apical furrows converging towards the external os (arrow).

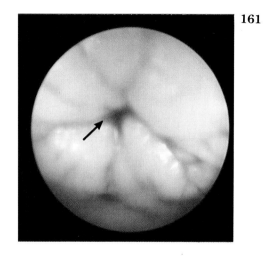

161

162 Vagina – early non-angular shrinkage period (mid pro-oestrus). The primary folds take on a greyish hue; they are less oedematous and their surface has a wrinkled appearance. The primary folds no longer fill the vaginal lumen (compare with **159**).

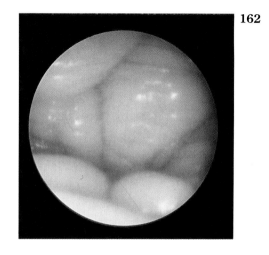

162

163 Vagina – early non-angular shrinkage period (mid pro-oestrus). The primary folds are less oedematous and are traversed by many secondary folds. The mucosa is beginning to lose its pink colour.

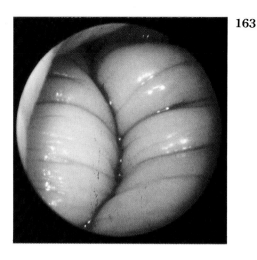

163

164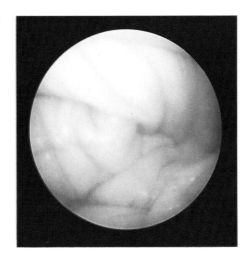

164 Vagina – obvious non-angular shrinkage period (late pro-oestrus). Lying obliquely across the receding primary folds, the secondary folds dominate the view. However, the profiles are still rounded. The mucosa has taken on a yellow colouration.

165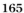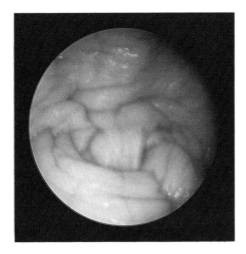

165 Vagina – advanced non-angular shrinkage period (late pro-oestrus). The secondary folds are convoluted and the mucosa is a creamy yellow colour. Some of the folds are becoming less rounded.

166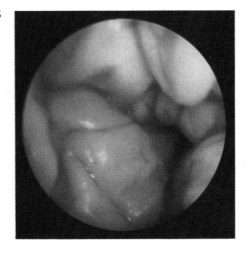

166 Vagina – early angular shrinkage period (early oestrus). The mucosa is thrown into irregular troughs and peaks, some of which are developing an angular profile.

167 Vagina – early angular shrinkage period (early oestrus). Low, crumpled folds of mucosa in the midvagina are beginning to develop sharp profiles.

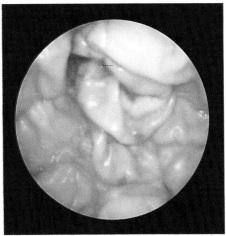

168 Vagina – obvious angular shrinkage period (standing oestrus). At the start of standing oestrus, many of the folds have developed angular peaks.

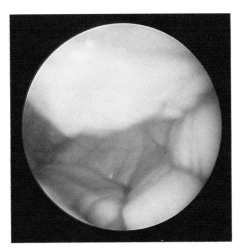

169 Caudal tubercle – obvious angular shrinkage period (standing oestrus). The caudal tubercle shows angulation and squaring of its profile.

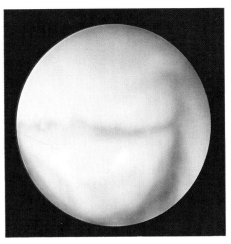

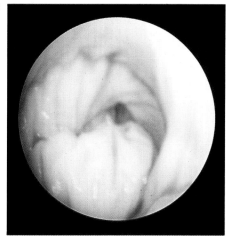

170 Vagina – maximum angular shrinkage period (standing oestrus). Sharp transverse ridges form a concertina pattern.

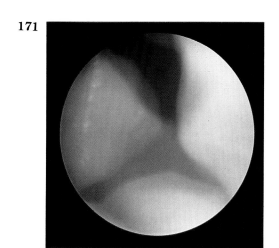

171 Vagina – maximum angular shrinkage period (standing oestrus). Another example of the sharply angled peaks. The slight haze at the bottom of the picture is postcoital fluid.

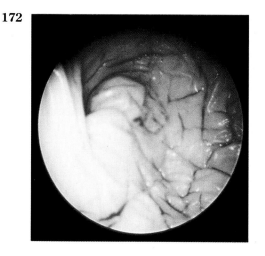

172 Vagina – late angular shrinkage period (end of standing oestrus). The peaks and trough are replaced by a 'crêpe paper' appearance. The mucosa is a pale yellow-pink and appears thin.

173   Vagina – obvious decline or cessation of shrinkage (late oestrus). The 'crêpe-paper' appearance has been replaced by low, rounded folds.

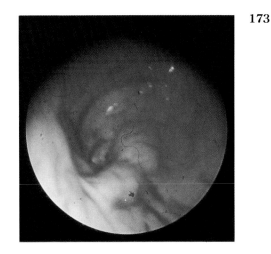

174   Vagina – metoestrus. The primary mucosal folds can be seen, but they are very much flattened. Strings of brown mucus are typical in early metoestrus.

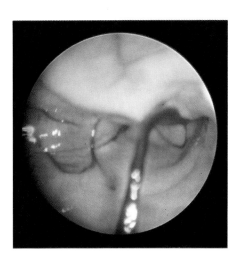

175   Vagina – metoestrus. In metoestrus the vaginal mucosa is reactive and tends to pucker into rosettes when touched with the endoscope.

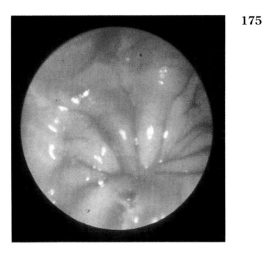

176

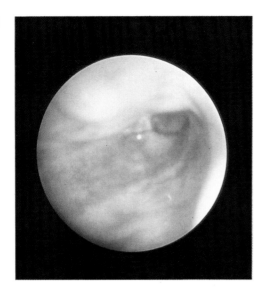

177

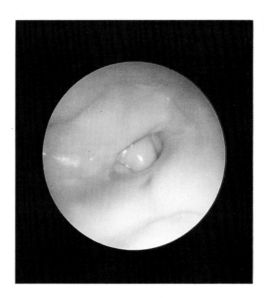

176 Vagina – anoestrus. Primary folds are just discernible. The mucosa is a patchy pink and yellow-pink colour. The paracervix can be seen above centre and to the right.

177 Paracervix – anoestrus. A close-up of the paracervix partially plugged by the caudal tubercle. Note the lack of folding of the cranial vaginal mucosa.

Abnormal vaginoscopic findings

178

179

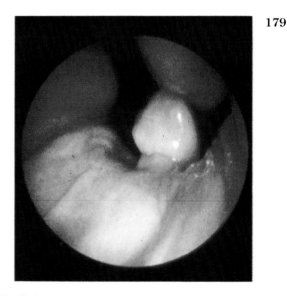

178 Pedunculated leiomyoma. Attached by a short pedicle (arrow) to the dorsal surface of the midvagina is an ovoid mass which is typical of an intravaginal leiomyoma. The paracervix and the caudal tubercle can be seen in the distance and to the left.

179 Polyp. There is a polyp at the vestibulovaginal junction. This was an incidental finding during a cyclic assessment.

8 Urethrocystoscopy

Introduction

The clinical signs of haematuria, dysuria, stranguria and increased frequency of urination are common to a number of disorders of the lower urinary tract, and further investigation is often required. Endoscopic examination of the lower urinary tract is indicated when a condition fails to respond to initial therapy, or when a tumour is suspected. Cystoscopy may also be employed for the investigation of incontinence, and is useful for the detection of ectopic ureters. For the investigation of bladder disorders, cystoscopy is at least complementary to radiography, and can provide additional information. Endoscopic biopsy enables confirmation of visual diagnoses.

The principal contraindication for urethrocystoscopy is acute bacterial infection, as the techniques employed may exacerbate the inflamed state.

Instruments and endoscopic procedure

Female dogs

The relatively straight and distensible urethra of the bitch enables the use of human cystoscopes. For most breeds, a standard adult cystoscope of 21 French (about 7 mm diameter) is adequate. Most manufacturers design rigid biopsy forceps for this size. For toy breeds, paediatric instruments may be required. As the bladder is pear-shaped in dogs, a forward- or slight oblique-viewing telescope is ideal for most work, although a 70° oblique telescope is useful for catheterisation of ureteric orifices.

General anaesthesia is required for the endoscopic procedure. The bitch is placed in dorsal recumbency at the end of the table, with the hind legs tied in a semiflexed position and abducted. The perineum, vulva and vestibule should be cleaned with a dilute aqueous solution of an antiseptic such as chlorhexidine gluconate. With the aid of a vaginal speculum, the urethral orifice on the ventral wall of the vestibule is located and the cystoscope sheath, with obturator, is then passed up the urethra. The introduction of the instrument may be facilitated by the prior dilatation of the urethra with bougies or an urethrotome; liberal use of aqueous jelly is essential. Once the instrument is within the bladder, the obturator is removed, allowing the urine to drain. The telescope is then locked into the sheath and the bladder is slowly filled with sterile saline, which distends the bladder and provides a good viewing medium.

Orientation points within the bladder are the cranial wall, the bladder neck, the ventral aspect of the bladder (uppermost as viewed with an air bubble introduced in the irrigating fluid) and the lateral walls on either side. The trigone and ureteric orifices are lowermost as viewed, and cranial to the bladder neck. Urine will be seen discharging in pulses from the ureteric orifices.

Biopsies of suspicious areas may be taken under visual control, but large blood vessels should be avoided. By draining some of the saline, the bladder can be partially deflated, thus minimising the risk of perforation. Although the biopsies obtained are small (about 3 mm in diameter), multiple samples may be taken with little increased risk. At the end of the examination, the saline should be drained before removing the sheath from the bladder; the urethra can be examined as the sheath is slowly withdrawn.

Male dogs

In male dogs the long arching course of the urethra does not permit rigid cystoscopy without resorting to either perineal urethrotomy or percutaneous perineal urethral puncture. Both of these are invasive techniques, the former being more so than the latter, but they do permit rigid cystoscopy in the manner described for the bitch.

As an alternative, fine flexible fibre-endoscopes may be used. The limiting factor is the internal diameter of the urethra, particularly in the region of the proximal os penis. Using a 3.5 mm broncho-fibrescope, most dogs over 15 kg can be examined.

Flexible cystoscopy in the male dog in most cases requires sedation only. The dog is restrained in right lateral recumbency, with the left leg semiabducted.

The penis is extruded and cleaned with a dilute antiseptic. The bladder is drained with a urinary catheter and partially filled with sterile saline. The saline is then drained and the bladder partially filled again. This washing is repeated until the drained fluid is clear. The bladder is then inflated with saline to provide a viewing medium.

Orientation with the flexible fibrescope is difficult. With the dog in left lateral recumbency, the air bubble will indicate the right lateral aspect. By retroflexing the endoscope off the cranial wall it is possible to look backwards and examine the bladder neck region. At the end of the procedure, the bladder should be drained of saline using a sterile urinary catheter.

Additional procedures

In human urology, endoscopic resection of bladder tumours is routinely performed. At present, the late stage at which most transitional cell carcinomas of dogs are detected precludes this mode of therapy.

However, with earlier diagnosis and assessment by cystoscopy, endoscopic resection may be used for the treatment of this type of tumour in dogs.

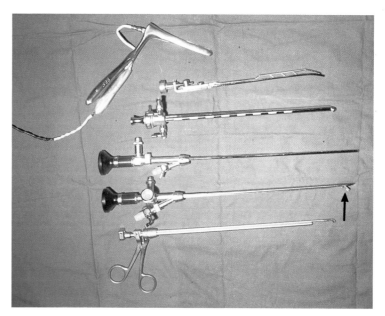

180

180 Instruments for rigid cystoscopy. (from top to bottom) vaginal speculum, urethral dilator (Otis urethrotome 10–30Fr), cystoscope sheath (21Fr), 12° fore-oblique telescope, 70° fore-oblique telescope with operating bridge (arrow), rigid biopsy forceps.

Normal endoscopic appearance

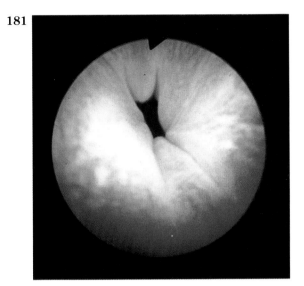

181 The female urethra. The urethra of the bitch is relatively short. Its luminal surface is thrown into longitudinal folds, and there are many large superficial blood vessels running along its length. The redness of the normal urethra, compared with that of the normal bladder, reflects the increased vascularity of the lamina propria.

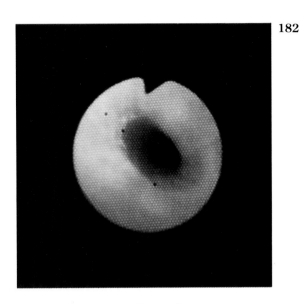

182 The male urethra. Except for numerous very small pits, the urethra in the male dog is relatively featureless for most of its length. In cross section, the urethral lumen varies from being circular to oval, and in the region of the os penis it may even be keyhole-shaped.

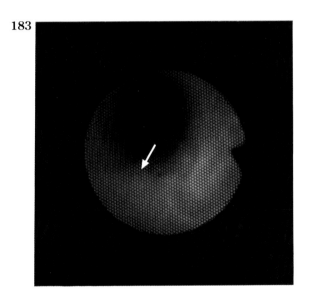

183 The prostatic urethra. The prostatic urethra is more dilated than the rest of the course, and has many ducts opening into it. On the ventral surface of the midprostatic region there is a discrete, oval mound, the verumontanum (arrow), where the vasa deferentia open.

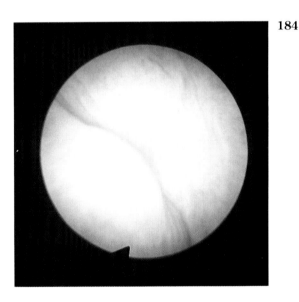

184 Fundus of a partially distended bladder. The appearance of the urothelium varies with the degree of distension of the bladder. The overall shape of the bladder tends to be distorted by adjacent abdominal viscera, and the urothelium is thrown into rugal folds. The vascular network is barely discernible.

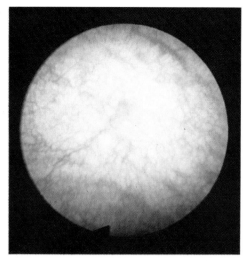

185   Fundus of a distended bladder. The urothelium becomes smooth and has a pale yellow-pink colour. The fine vascular network is readily discernible.

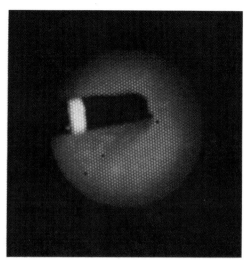

186   The bladder neck. With a flexible endoscope it is possible to examine the neck region of the bladder by retroflexion. Here, the endoscope is seen entering the bladder.

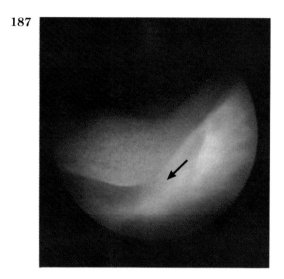

187   The ureteric orifice. The ureteric orifices vary in shape from low, slanting, horseshoe-shaped arches, as seen here, to short, oval slits on low papillae. The orifices are usually symmetrical in position and shape, although, occasionally, one of the orifices may be more caudally placed. Urine (arrow) will be seen discharging in pulses from the orifices, reflecting the peristaltic nature of the ureters.

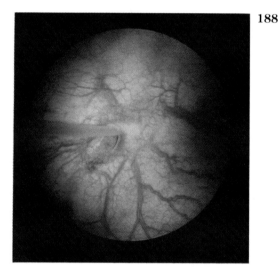

188   Ureteric catheterisation. Once the ureteric orifice has been located, the ureter may be catheterised; a 70° telescope with an operating bridge assists this procedure. Ureteric catheterisation permits retrograde contrast radiography or the sampling of urine from each kidney for bacteriology, for the assessment of individual renal function or for cytology. Note the large blood vessels radiating from around the ureteric orifice.

Abnormal endoscopic features

189

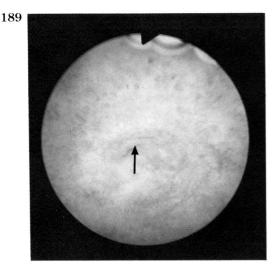

190

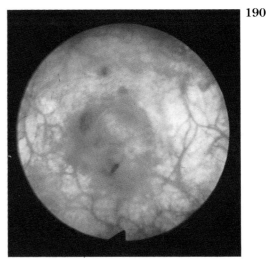

189 Urachal remnant – congenital abnormality. A small, pit-like depression (arrow) can be seen in the centre of relatively normal urothelium in the cranioventral region of the bladder. This urachal remnant is 1–2 mm in diameter and has no associated pathological changes. In this case, the defect was an incidental finding. Note the silvery hemispheres at the top of the picture – these are air bubbles which collect at the highest point in the bladder. As the dog is in dorsal recumbency, this is the ventral aspect of the bladder.

190 Infected urachal remnant. The urachal remnant (centre) may act as a nidus for chronic infection. A moderate **degree** of erythema, with loss of normal vascular pattern over the immediate area of 1–3 cm diameter, can be seen. A cobblestone-like surface, which can progress to nodular hyperplasia (see **204**), may be a further variation. A chronically infected urachal remnant may act as a focus of bacteria that is not easily eliminated by antibiotic therapy and which may require surgical ablation.

191

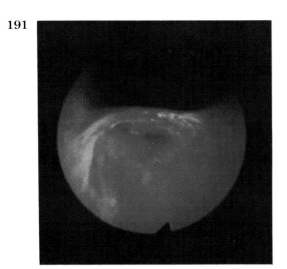

192

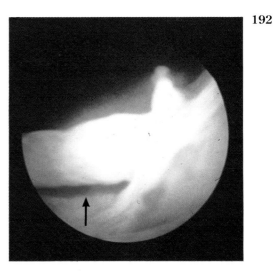

191 Ectopic ureters. In the centre of the picture an ectopic ureteric orifice can be discerned as a slit beneath a flap-like structure on the dorsal wall of the proximal urethra; urine was seen to discharge from it. The erythematous and haemorrhagic appearance of the flap was due to minor trauma by the cystoscope. In the distance is the bladder neck.

192 Transplanted ureteric orifice. Following reimplantation of an ectopic ureter, the neo-orifice may be checked by cystoscopy. Here, the new orifice (arrow) shows no signs of stricture, and urine was seen discharging. In this case, a suture (yellow and blurred) (5/0 Dexon™, Davis and Geck, UK) is still present five weeks after the operation.

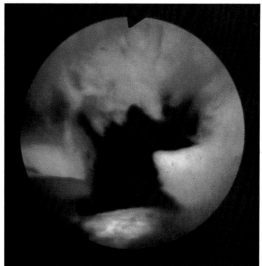

193 Transitional cell carcinoma. The normal, smooth circle of the internal aspect of the bladder neck has been replaced by irregular and ragged tissue. There is evidence of haemorrhage and of necrotic tissue (yellow plaque, bottom of picture). A biopsy confirmed the malignant nature of this lesion.

The overall appearance of transitional cell carcinomas varies according to the site and the extent of the tumour. Most cases have fine, vascular, papillary fronds, seen either as a diffuse lesion encircling the bladder neck region, or as large and often multiple masses. Moss-like plaques, indicating areas of carcinoma *in situ,* may be seen at the periphery of larger tumours, or as discrete islands elsewhere.

194

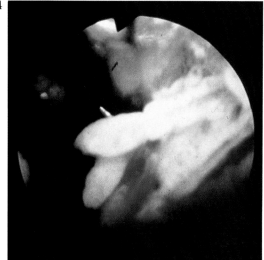

194 Transitional cell carcinoma – papillary fronds. The finger-like projections with a central vascular core are characteristic macroscopic findings of a transitional cell carcinoma. Each of the projections is about 1 mm across.

Papillary tumours are highly vascular and friable. They bleed readily, making the viewing medium turbid. Biopsies should, therefore, be taken at the completion of the visual examination.

195

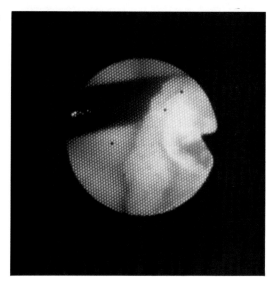

195 Rhabdomyosarcoma. A multilobular mass can be seen adjacent to the flexible endoscope as it enters the bladder. (Compare with **186**) The surface of the lobules is relatively smooth and featureless, except for fine, traversing blood vessels. Histopathology showed this to be a rhabdomyosarcoma of the bladder, a rare tumour that affects young and, predominantly, male dogs. The tumour usually arises from the trigone region and tends to obscure the ureteric orifices.

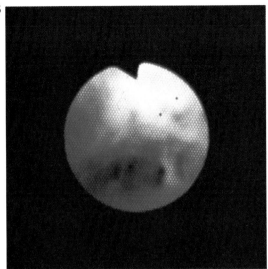

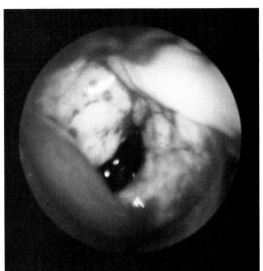

196   Prostatic carcinoma. The lumen of the prostatic urethra is irregular in cross section and is traversed by fibrinous tags. Cytological examination of a washing from this area demonstrated malignant epithelial cells. The dog had a prostatic adenocarcinoma.

The endoscopic appearance of a prostatic malignancy will vary from case to case. Where invasion has occurred, the prostatic urethra becomes indistensible and narrowed such that the flexible endoscope cannot be advanced, as in the case illustrated here. However, where the urethra is not invaded, the endoscopic appearance may be normal.

197   Urethral tumours. At this midregion of the urethra, most of the luminal aspect is replaced by a white, smooth, multilobulated annular mass with areas of superficial haemorrhage. The lumen is blocked by a blood clot. A biopsy and, later, postmortem samples, confirmed the malignant nature of this lesion.

Urethral carcinomas and eroding sarcomas may also develop as florid, partially ulcerated, necrotic areas with papillary fingers. Urethral carcinomas may be continuous with a bladder transitional cell carcinoma or a solitary lesion.

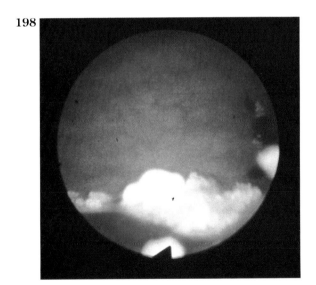

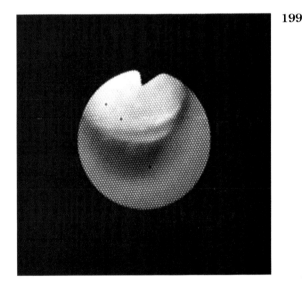

198 & 199   Urolithiasis. Calculi appear as white, round or oval masses of varying size that lie in the dependent portion of the bladder. In male dogs (**199**) calculi may be seen in the urethra, proximal to the os penis as the flexible endoscope is introduced; they may be pushed back into the bladder to join other stones. In all cases of urolithiasis the bladder urothelium will be hyperaemic, reflecting the concurrent cystitis.

In female dogs, and male dogs with previously performed high perineal urethrostomies, the calculi may be removed through the sheath either by physical flushing or with forceps. Large calculi may first require fragmentation either with crushing forceps or by electrohydraulic lithotripsy.

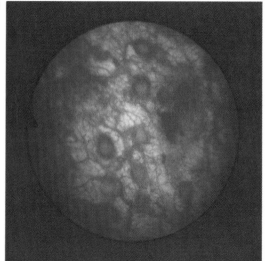

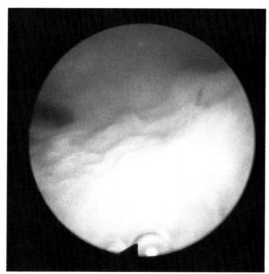

200 Bacterial cystitis. The cystoscopic appearance suggestive of acute cystitis is one of patchy or generalised hyperaemia and erythema. In this case, multiple small (1–2 mm diameter) lesions resembling pustules can be seen. Note the erythematous halo surrounding the yellow-white plaques.

Occasionally, small areas of petechiation will be seen and the urothelium will have a tendency to bleed readily.

201 Chronic cystitis. Chronic cystitis is seen more commonly than acute cystitis, as a secondary condition. Hyperaemia and erythema are the usual features, but the urothelium may also have a general, ragged, fimbriated appearance. Mineral deposits, recognised as white flecking on the surface, are another indicator of the chronic nature of the condition.

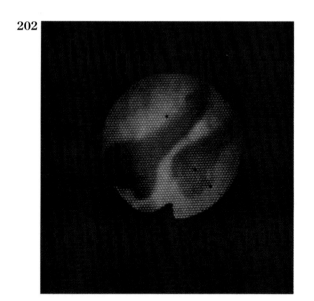

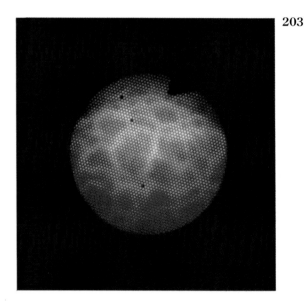

202 Polypoid cystitis. Two club-shaped masses, one a dark red and the other more blue, can be seen lying across a relatively normal urothelium. These polyps were about 3 cm in length and arose from the ventral aspect of the bladder. Polypoid cystitis is a proliferative condition of the bladder that is usually induced by chronic irritation.

203 Cystitis cystica. This mulberry-like mass was seen to the right of the midline in a dog with chronic cystitis due to urolithiasis. The mass was about 2 cm in diameter, slightly erythematous and multilobulated. Following excision, it was found to be non-neoplastic, but it resembled cystitis cystica with von Brunn's nests. These two bizarre hyperplastic conditions are induced by chronic irritation.

204 Nodular hyperplasia. Projecting from the cranio-ventral region of the bladder, an erythematous partially lobulated mass can be seen. Biopsy of the mass showed it to be hyperplastic and inflammatory in nature, and not neoplastic.

Nodular hyperplasia is another chronic inflammatory condition that causes mild, but intractable, cystitis-like signs. Most frequently seen in the cranioventral region of the bladder, the condition is thought to be associated with a chronic, low-grade, local infection of a urachal remnant. Treatment consists of a prolonged course of antibiotics, and surgical excision may be required.

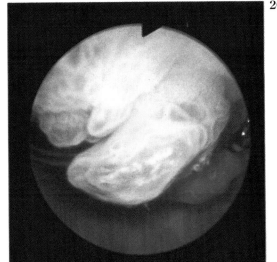

205 Cyclophosphamide-induced cystitis. Most of this field shows generalised erythema, with an area of haemorrhage and fibrinous tags (arrow). This is typical of the severe sterile cystitis induced by acrolin, a metabolite of cyclophosphamide excreted in the urine.

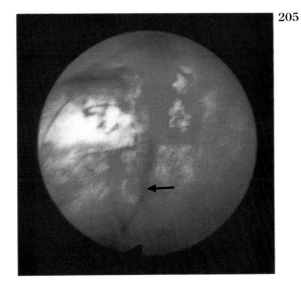

206 Cyclophosphamide-induced necrotising cystitis. In this view of a partially inflated bladder, most of the urothelium is markedly erythematous and haemorrhagic. The white-green ovoid area (above centre) is an ulcer, 2–3 cm in diameter, occupying most of the cranioventral aspect of the bladder. The dog had been on adjuvant cyclophosphamide therapy for several months prior to examination. The condition spontaneously resolved several months later.

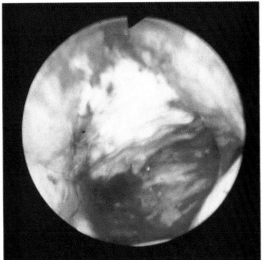

207

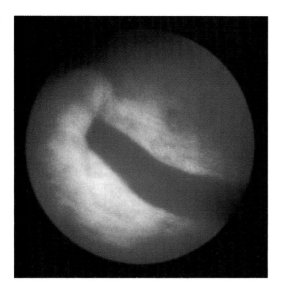

207 Haematuria of renal origin. Cystoscopy may also be used to collect urine from each kidney separately, following ureteric catheterisation. Indications vary, but in this case the urine discharging from the right ureteric orifice was a dark brown-red colour, whereas that from the left was pale yellow. The right ureter was catheterised and a sample of the urine was collected for laboratory examination. Cytology revealed a few apparently normal cells. The brown colouration was attributed to the presence of changed haemoglobin rather than to erythrocytes. Although no obvious injuries had been noticed at the time, the dog had developed haematuria after being hit by a car. It was concluded that there was an organising renal haematoma. (The overall redness of the view is a photographic artefact.)

9 Laparoscopy

Introduction

Laparoscopy permits direct visual examination of the abdominal viscera by a relatively simple, quick and minimally traumatic procedure. It also enables visually selected biopsies to be obtained without major surgery. This chapter considers laparoscopy in the dog and cat; other species are discussed in subsequent chapters.

The indications for laparoscopy are similar to those for exploratory laparotomy:

• Direct visual examination of the various abdominal structures including the peritoneum, diaphragm, liver, gallbladder, kidney, spleen, pancreas, ovaries, urinary bladder (external), stomach and intestines (external).

• Biopsy under direct visual control to obtain samples for histopathological diagnosis and other laboratory tests.

• Aspiration of bile from the gallbladder.

• Injection of positive contrast agents into the gallbladder or spleen (for contrast radiography).

The principal contraindications for laparoscopy are:

• Diaphragmatic rupture.

• Peritonitis.

• Intra-abdominal adhesions.

• Advanced cardiac failure.

• Coagulopathy.

Laparotomy may be preferable to laparoscopy if any of the differential diagnoses require surgical intervention.

Choice of instruments

Laparoscope

Rigid endoscopes are used for laparoscopy. A range of sizes from 2.7–10 mm diameter is available. The larger diameter telescopes provide a better field of view, while the narrow instruments cause least trauma. A 5 mm diameter telescope is suitable for most cases but one of 2.7 mm may be required for cats and toy breeds of dogs. Fore-oblique (25–30° from straight ahead) viewing telescopes are the most suitable for the majority of situations. Operating laparoscopes are available, but accessory instruments via a second puncture are preferable.

Accessory instruments

Biopsies may be obtained with a variety of instruments including a Menghini aspiration needle, Tru-Cut™ (Travenol, UK & USA) biopsy needle, and purpose-designed biopsy forceps with an electrocoagulation facility.

Trocar and cannula

The laparoscope and accessory instruments are introduced into the abdominal cavity through separate cannulae with gas-tight seals.

Insufflation equipment

Intra-abdominal gas (pneumoperitoneum) is essential in order to perform laparoscopy in mammals. Gas is introduced into the abdomen through a special blunt-tipped needle: a Verres cannula, 10 cm in length, is adequate in both the dog and the cat.

Gas may be introduced manually with a large syringe via a three-way tap. However, with this method the assessment of intra-abdominal gas pressure is subjective, and frequent replenishment is required.

An automatic system is preferable, as this maintains the intra-abdominal gas pressure at a set value of about 10 mmHg. Automatic insufflators display the intra-abdominal gas pressure, the gas flow rate and the total gas volume.

The choice of gas is important: air should be avoided as fatal air-emboli may be produced. Either carbon dioxide or nitrous oxide can be used safely, as both are absorbed from the peritoneal cavity.

Technique

Preparation

Although sedation and local analagesia may be sufficient on rare occasions, general anaesthesia is usually required. The urinary bladder should be emptied to avoid inadvertent puncture by a trocar. The animal should be secured in either dorsal or lateral recum-bency, and the area(s) of the puncture site(s) should be clipped and prepared as for surgery. Asepsis should be maintained and the instruments must be sterilised before use.

Puncture sites for laparoscopy in the dog or cat

The midline approach has the advantage over the lateral method, since the whole of the abdominal cavity may be examined. However, in obese patients the falciform fat may obscure vision, making the lateral approach preferable. For the latter, the upper-most sublumbar fossa is used for all punctures.

When using a ventral midline approach, the sites for puncture are:

- **Verres cannula** – lateral and caudal to the umbilicus to avoid the fatty falciform ligament, liver and spleen.

- **Laparoscope and accessory instruments** – lateral to the midline between the xiphoid process and the umbilicus.

For right-handed operators, the accessory instruments should be introduced to the right of the laparoscope to allow manipulation by the right hand.

Pneumoperitoneum

It is most important that pneumoperitoneum is established before trocarisation for the instruments. The Verres cannula is introduced through a small skin incision. To check correct positioning, a test injection of saline, together with aspiration, should be performed; if blood or urine is obtained, the needle should be repositioned. In animals with ascites, the transudate should be partially drained. Overinsufflation is potentially hazardous to the patient, as the venous return to the heart will be compromised and gas emboli may be induced.

Laparoscope and accessory instruments

Once pneumoperitoneum is achieved, the trocar and cannula may be inserted. Again, a small skin incision is made and the trocar and cannula are introduced by firm but controlled pressure. A stabbing motion should never be used. As soon as the abdomen is penetrated, the trocar is withdrawn to prevent damage to internal organs from the sharp point. If the cannula is correctly positioned, gas may be freely aspirated from the peritoneal cavity.

Orientation within the abdomen

As with exploratory laparotomy, a systematic examination of the entire abdominal contents should always be performed. For such an examination to be effective, a working knowledge of the anatomy is necessary. It may be helpful to divide the abdomen into quadrants.

Fogging and fluid on the objective may be remedied by gentle rubbing on the omentum. The tip of the accessory instrument may prove difficult to locate, but the telescope and instrument can be brought into contact by external manipulation. A blunt accessory instrument may be used for lifting and moving loops of bowel and mesentery. Ballooning of the omentum can be counteracted with a rowing motion of the accessory instrument or Verres cannula.

End of procedure

Once the examination is complete, the cannulae may be removed. First the Verres cannula is withdrawn, then the accessory and, last, that for the laparoscope. The intra-abdominal gas pressure should be relieved through this last cannula. The abdominal wall punctures for the laparoscope, accessory cannulae and all skin incisions should be sutured.

Laparoscopic appearance

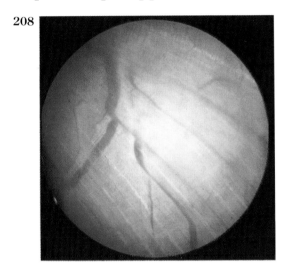

208

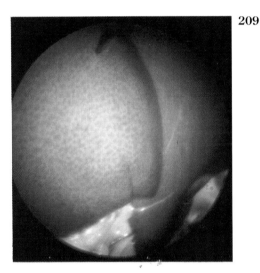

209

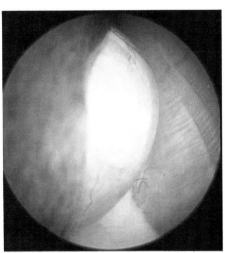

210

208 Diaphragm – dog. The muscle bundles are aligned parallel to the radius of the diaphragm, and are interspaced by fibrous bands. A variety of sizes of blood vessels can be seen crossing the diaphragm in a branching network.

209 Liver – dog. The liver is a deep red-brown colour with a smooth surface and sharp borders. Here, the liver has a rather more marked portal pattern than is usually seen. A small portion of mesentery can be seen at the bottom of the picture.

210 Liver, gallbladder, diaphragm – dog. The pale blue gallbladder can be seen protruding from between the lobes of the liver and silhouetted against the diaphragm.

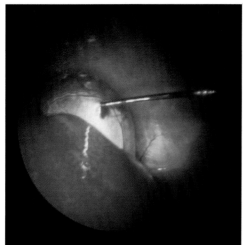

211 Gallbladder aspiration. Under endoscopic direction, the gallbladder can be punctured with the tip of a long needle (e.g., a 20G spinal needle, 10 cm long). Bile is aspirated into a syringe and can be submitted for cytological and bacteriological examination. By injecting a radiopaque, iodinated contrast agent (5–10 ml) the extrahepatic biliary system can be evaluated radiographically.

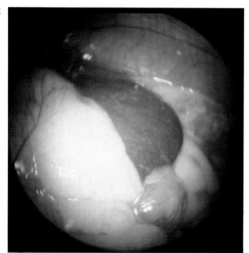

212 Spleen – cat. The spleen is a dark red-purple colour. The margins tend to be less acute than those of the liver, and the surface is textured. Lying above the spleen is a section of intestine, and to the left and below is mesenteric fat.

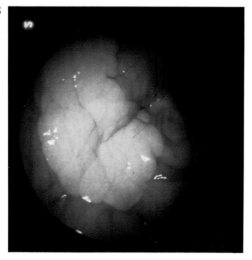

213 Pancreas – dog. The normal pancreas appears as an oblong, multilobulated structure that is pale cream in colour. The right arm lies in close proximity to the duodenum, but the left is less easily visualised as it tends to be lost in the surrounding structures.

214 Kidney – cat. The kidney can be visualised through the renal capsule (note the capsular blood vessels). The fibrous capsule adds a silvery grey sheen to the kidney. Here, the kidney is being manoeuvred with a blunt probe, but this demonstrates in principle how endoscopic-directed biopsy with a Tru-cut™ needle can be performed. Visualisation of the kidney facilitates both the accurate biopsy of focal renal lesions and the assessment of post-biopsy haemorrhage.

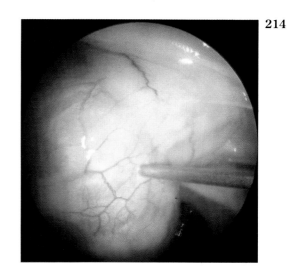

215 Uterine horn and ovarian bursa – dog. The uterine horn can be seen as the pale pink tubular structure traversing from the left to the centre of the view, towards an ovoid yellow mass, the fat-laden ovarian bursa. The kidney can be seen below and behind the ovarian bursa.

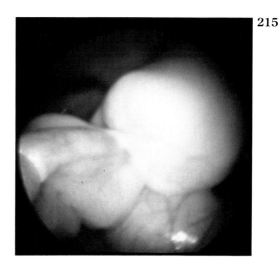

216 Small intestine – dog. The external surface of the various parts of the intestinal tract can be viewed by laparoscopy. It is, however, difficult to follow a portion for any distance because of the convoluted nature of the intestines and the overlying mesentery.

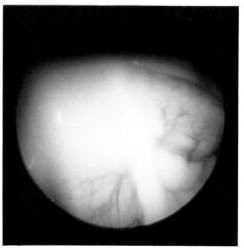

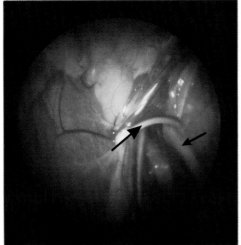

217 **Inguinal ring (internal aspect) – male dog.** The abdominal muscle wall (pink) can be seen on the left and a small portion of the urinary bladder (grey) is visible on the right. The vas deferens (large arrow) crosses the centre of the field from left to right. It appears as a pale cream, arched structure, running from the inguinal ring to tuck in between the ureter (small arrow) and the bladder.

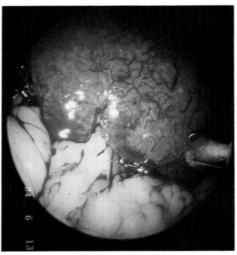

218 **Liver biopsy – cholangiohepatitis in a cat.** The liver is markedly abnormal. Note the pale colour and the congested, tortuous blood vessels. On the right of the field the biopsy forceps can be seen. The biopsy site is the V-shaped indentation on the border of the lobe in the centre of the picture. There is minimal bleeding.

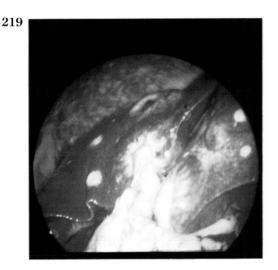

219 **Metastatic deposits within the liver – dog.** Much of the liver appears normal, that is, it has a smooth surface and sharp borders, but there are multiple, pale, discrete masses protruding from the parenchyma, several of which have characteristic central depressions. The primary tumour was found to be a pancreatic adenocarcinoma. (The overall yellow tone is a photographic artefact.)

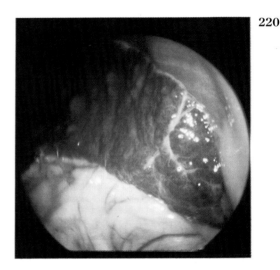

220 **Cirrhosis with nodular regeneration of the liver – dog.** The liver has a shrunken appearance with an irregular 'cobblestone' surface and white fibrous tracts. Multiple, lighter coloured nodules are present, representing areas of active regeneration.

10 Canine arthroscopy

Introduction

Most arthroscopies in the dog are performed for diagnostic reasons, but surgical arthroscopic procedures have been described for the hip joint, for the repair of ruptured cranial cruciate ligaments and for the treatment of osteochondritis dissecans of the shoulder. Arthroscopy undoubtedly has an important role in the future of veterinary rheumatology, but the technique is currently too specialised and expensive to merit routine application in general small animal practice.

There are a number of indications for arthroscopy:

- As an adjunct to clinical and radiological investigations, when the presenting problem does not warrant full arthrotomy.

- To facilitate preoperative planning, ahead of a proposed arthrotomy. Postoperative arthroscopies can be used to evaluate the results of surgery and to investigate surgical failures.

- To perform surgery on intra-articular structures, rapidly, under direct visualisation, with nominal invasion of tissues and minimum associated morbidity. In particular, arthroscopy is a useful way to obtain biopsies of synovial membrane.

- To monitor the progress of chronic arthritic disorders by sequential arthroscopies.

Arthroscopy is contraindicated in the following circumstances:

- Arthroscopic examination through infected, abraded or otherwise damaged skin can lead to septic arthritis because bacteria can be inoculated directly into the joint space.

- Joint infection is a relative contraindication. Treatment regimes for septic arthritis may include arthroscopic lavage.

Choice of instrument

Endoscopes of less than 3 mm overall diameter are required for arthroscopy in dogs. Telescopes of 1.7 mm and 2.2 mm diameter are available requiring insertion cannulae of 2 mm and 3 mm diameter respectively. A sharp trocar and a blunt obturator are used with the cannula. A second cannula is needed if endoscopic-guided biopsy is to be performed. When not in use, the telescope should be stored in a protective sleeve to prevent damage to this fragile instrument.

Technique

It is beyond the scope of this text to provide detailed descriptions of arthroscopic approaches to specific joints, but general principles are discussed.

The patient is anaesthetised and full aseptic precautions are maintained throughout the procedure. Following aspiration of the synovial fluid, the joint is dilated by infusing 10–30 ml of sterile saline. A Teflon catheter is inserted into the distended joint and connected to a bag of isotonic saline to establish continuous fluid inflow. A 20 ml or 50 ml syringe, connected to the infusion system by a three-way tap, can be used intermittently to flush and distend the joint with additional sterile saline.

A stab incision is made in the skin overlying the distended joint, and a sharp trocar, ensheathed in a steel cannula, is used to enter the joint capsule. The sharp point of the trocar may damage intra-articular structures as the instrument is manoeuvred within the joint space, so it is replaced by a blunt obturator. Once the instrument is in position, the obturator is removed and the joint is flushed thoroughly to remove blood and debris, before it is distended again with sterile saline. The viewing telescope is inserted into the cannula, which protects its delicate optical structures and also functions as an outflow port for waste fluid. For surgical arthroscopies, two or three cannulae must be inserted to accommodate instruments in addition to the viewing telescope. To reduce the risk of damaging the viewing telescope or surgical instruments, major manipulations are always performed with the obturator in the cannula. On completion of the procedure, the joint is flushed thoroughly and the skin incisions are closed with a single suture.

Arthroscopy is associated with few important complications. Subcutaneous swelling may temporarily occur as a result of leakage from the breached synovium, but it is usually inconsequential. There are no data for dogs, but in humans, other complications have been documented including tender postoperative scar (14%), joint effusion and haemarthrosis (9%), hypoaesthaesia distal to the entry portal (0.4%), non-pyogenic joint inflammation (0.3%), joint infection (0.07%) and granuloma (0.03%).

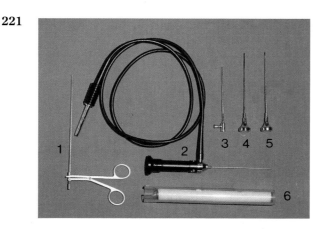

221

221 Arthroscopic equipment. Biopsy forceps (1), Telescope and light guide (2), Cannula (3), Obturator (4), Trocar (5), Protective storage sheath (6).

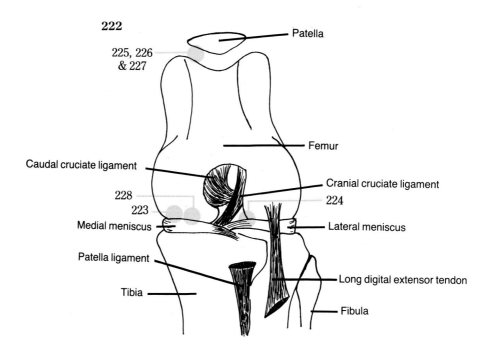

222

222 Flexed stifle joint. A schematic cranial aspect of the flexed stifle joint of the dog, mapping the areas illustrated by the arthroscopic photographs (**223–228**).

223 Medial meniscus. The middle and caudal portions of the meniscus lie between the medial femoral condyle (top) and the articular surface of the tibia below. Whisps of pink, translucent synovial villi (arrow) cross the joint cavity.

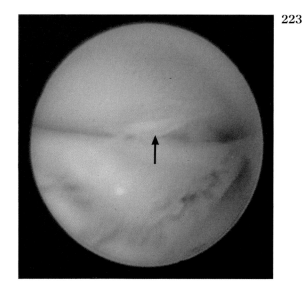

224 Lateral meniscus. The lateral femoral condyle can be seen at the top of the field. The lower two-thirds show the lateral meniscus with its sharply concaved inner margin adjacent to the intercondylar eminence (arrow) of the tibia.

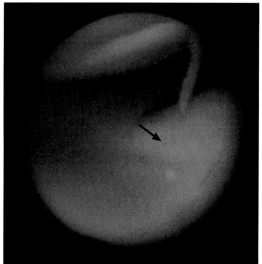

225 Femoropatellar joint. The trochlear groove of the femur occupies the lower field of view. Above is the patella (top left) and part of the fat pad (top right). Synovial villi cross immediately below the patella.

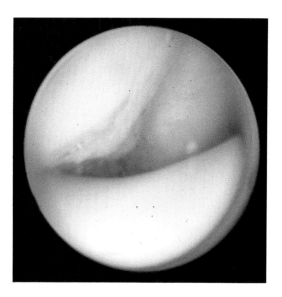

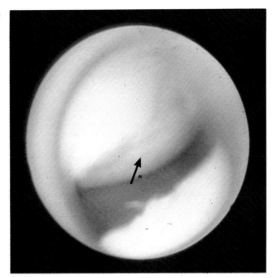

226 **Degenerative joint disease – femoropatellar joint.** A similar view to that shown in **225**, but note the area of roughness, dullness and flatness (arrow) adjacent to the joint cavity on the lower aspect of the patella. The femoral condyle has a markedly ragged skyline. This appearance is indicative of articular cartilage degeneration.

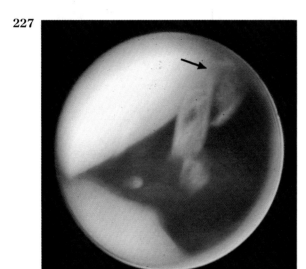

227 **Degenerative joint disease – femoropatellar joint.** The patella (top left) has an area of roughness (arrow) with flakes of cartilage projecting into the joint cavity.

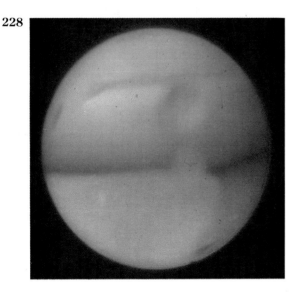

228 **Medial femoral condyle with ulcer.** The medial femoral condyle shows an ulcer in the articular cartilage. The medial meniscus (left of centre) is somewhat rounded in profile. A diagnosis of degenerative joint disease is warranted.

11 Avian endoscopy

Endoscopic examination of birds is a well established technique and can be used in individuals of different species and sizes. The use of an endoscope to sex birds, or to study their gonads, was first carried out by field biologists many years ago and has become a recognised procedure in research, as well as in avicultural medicine. It should be mentioned, however, that other, less invasive methods of sexing certain birds have found favour in recent years, for example, external measurements, examination of the feathers, cloacoscopy, or chromosomal techniques.

The main indications for endoscopy in birds are as follows:

● **Sex determination of monomorphic species.** Direct visual inspection of the gonads provides information on sexual activity, reproductive performance and age of the bird, these being manifested by the size, shape, colour and vascularisation of the gonad. Normal development of the gonads of the barn owl (*Tyto alba*) is illustrated in **229**. 'Laparoscopic' examination of birds is facilitated by the fact that insufflation of the body cavity is not required: the air sacs provide an already air-filled chamber.

● **Clinical diagnosis.** Techniques for clinical diagnosis are based on direct visual inspection of the body cavities and organs. There are many examples in avian work: external auditory canal (auroscopy or otoscopy), nasal cavities (rhinoscopy), cranial sinuses, pharynx (pharyngoscopy), trachea (tracheoscopy), oesophagus (oesophagoscopy), crop (ingluvioscopy), gizzard (gastroscopy), coelomic cavity (coeloscopy — commonly called 'laparoscopy').

In addition to permitting or facilitating the viewing of structure, endoscopy allows samples to be taken (endoscopic biopsy) and operative procedures to be performed (endoscopic surgery).

229

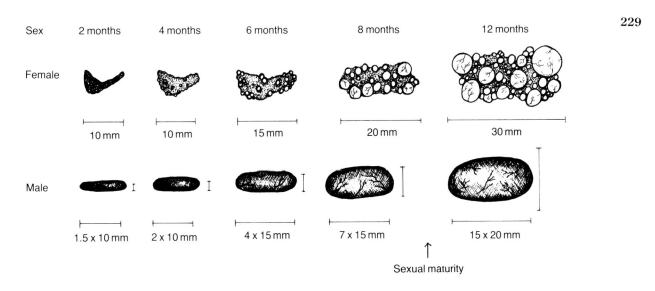

229 Developmental changes in the gonads of the barn owl (*Tyto alba*).

Contraindications

Some veterinary surgeons remain reluctant to use anaesthetics in birds on the grounds that avian patients are 'high anaesthetic risks', but this is not necessarily true. With good anaesthetic technique and perioperative care, a mortality rate of less than 0.1% can be achieved. However, a higher mortality rate (up to 2%), may occur when examining old and fat birds, especially birds of prey and parrots.

At postmortem examination, fatalities that have occurred after laparoscopy (coeloscopy) include aspergillosis, tuberculosis, cardiovascular conditions (mainly fatty change and arteriosclerosis) and visceral gout. Inhalation pneumonia occurs if the birds have not been deprived of water, or because of ptyalism (inhalation of saliva). It is possible that larger members of the orders Ciconiiformes (storks) and Falconiformes (hawks, falcons etc.) are particularly susceptible. Preoperative fasting is important in such large species: if it is not performed, puncturing of the enlarged digestive tract, and especially the gizzard, can occur.

Choice of instruments

For coeloscopy, it is best to use forward-viewing telescopes, the diameter of which will vary according to the size of the patient:

● Needlescopes (1.5–1.8 mm external diameter, 150 mm long) for birds weighing 30–150 g.

● Arthroscopes (2.8–3 mm external diameter, 150 mm long) for birds weighing 150–2000 g.

● Laparoscopes (4–5 mm external diameter, 300 mm long) for birds weighing over 2000 g.

The choice of instrument for other techniques will depend upon the species of bird, the structure to be investigated and the facilities available.

Technique for coeloscopic (laparoscopic) sex determination

For small birds (under 250 g in weight), it is advisable to use a small 'operating table': suitable dimensions are 250 mm by 150 mm, and 100 mm high. The table should be perspex, with aluminium sides that can be moulded to the shape of the bird. A heating pad is placed underneath the operating table, providing a temperature of 28°C.

The table is useful for two reasons:

● Hypothermia and hyperthermia are avoided. An optimum temperature is maintained throughout the operating procedure, and direct contact with the heating pad, which can sometimes cause overheating, is avoided.

● Positioning of the anaesthetised bird is facilitated.

The subject is positioned in right lateral recumbency with the wings folded in the normal anatomical position, or, if the bird is anaesthetised, the left wing is held clear of the operation site. The left leg is fully extended cranially and secured. For many birds, the optimum surgical site is the upper part of the triangle formed by the cranial edge of the pubis, the proximal part of the femur, and the last rib (**230**). An alternative technique is to extend the left leg caudally and to insert the endoscope between the ultimate and penultimate ribs (**237**). Other methods of gaining access to the body cavity are discussed on p. 100.

Once a few feathers have been plucked from the surgical site and the area has been cleaned with antiseptic solution, a small incision (of the same size as the diameter of the telescope to be used) is made with a sharp pair of scissors. The trocar and cannula are then inserted into the cavity. The instruments are directed upwards (dorsally) at an angle of 45° to the abdominal wall. If these guidelines are not followed, beginners may puncture a vital organ (usually the liver or gizzard). Blunt-ended trocars are recommended rather than sharp ones.

It may be considered bad practice to introduce the telescope through the abdominal wall without a cannula because the very fragile lens and its seal at the tip of the telescope can suffer serious damage. In addition, the cannula facilitates the withdrawal and further introduction of the telescope, for example, after cleaning. However, the cannula can be a disadvantage because it unnecessarily increases the size of the incision that must be made. To illustrate, it is worth noting that a 2.7 mm diameter endoscope **without** a cannula gives a better view and is almost as small as a 1.7 mm instrument with a cannula.

If the endoscope is positioned correctly, the operator

should be able to see cranially the wall of the right air sac, the lung and a small part of the liver and the gizzard to the left (**231**). When carrying out surgical sexing, the first structure that should be identified is the anterior (cranial) lobe of the kidney. The gonad, together with the adrenal gland, is to be found at the cranioventral edge of the kidney. In small birds it is often unnecessary to puncture the wall of the right air sac, since the normal wall is transparent and the gonads can be seen by pressing the tip of the telescope on the wall. In larger species, however, this may not be a reliable method. Sometimes, particularly in obese birds, fat deposits obscure the view, in which case the air sac wall has to be punctured. Such an incision heals rapidly (probably within a few hours), while muscle and skin sutures take 3–7 days.

Although the basic internal anatomy of birds varies very little, there are differences in body shape and size, and the operator may be confused if these are not taken into account. Differences also occur in the reproductive tract that relate to age, species and season of the year. As a general rule, coeloscopy for sex determination is best performed at the beginning or the end of the breeding season.

230

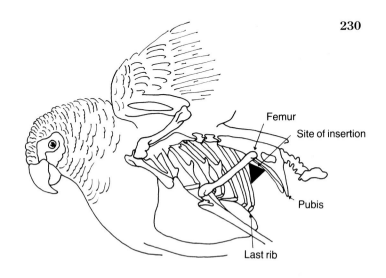

230 Surgical site for sex determination in a psittacine bird.

231

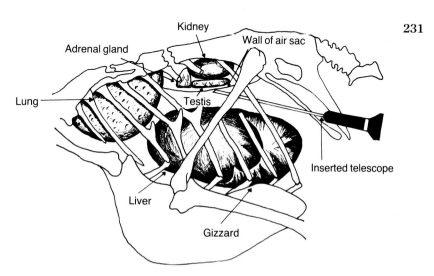

231 Relative positions of organs during sex determination.

Techniques for clinical diagnosis

Techniques for clinical diagnosis differ little from those described for mammals elsewhere in this Atlas. There are certain anatomical features of birds that make them ideal subjects for endoscopic investigation, for example, the presence of air sacs, a cloaca and, in most species, a crop. The particular relevance of these features to endoscopy is shown in **Table 2** on p. 112.

Endoscopic examination of the upper alimentary tract is particularly useful in birds, and can be performed using rigid or flexible instruments (**232 & 236**). Cloacal examination is also important. The anatomy of the cloaca is shown in **269 & 270**, p. 115.

Battery-operated endoscopes are useful in birds, especially to examine orifices. For example, one significant feature of an auriscope is that the speculum permits the entry of air. This can be advantageous when examining the upper alimentary/respiratory tracts, but it can cause complications during coeloscopy if gaseous anaesthesia is being employed.

It should be noted that various routes can be used to enter and examine the body cavity for diagnostic purposes. These can be summarised as follows:

- Behind the last rib.

- Between the penultimate and last ribs.

- Via the sternal notch.

- Dorsal to the pubic bone and caudal to the ischium.

- Ventral midline, immediately caudal to the sternum (direct access to liver).

- Unpaired interclavicular air sac. Minor surgery is needed (access to upper respiratory tract, thyroid, oesophagus etc.).

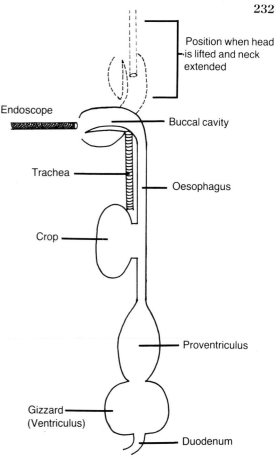

232 Diagrammatic representation of the upper alimentary tract of a bird, showing the various structures that can be examined endoscopically. Note the importance of raising the bird's head, and straightening the neck, if the instrument is to be passed further than the pharynx.

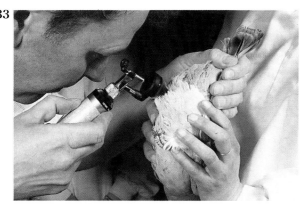

233 Examination of the cloaca of a pigeon (*Columba livia*), using an auriscope (otoscope). Simple endoscopes are of great value in birds.

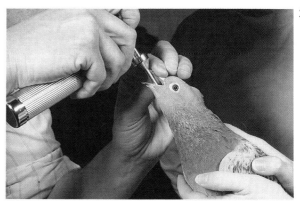

234 Examination of the oesophagus and crop of a pigeon. In this case the instrument is battery-operated, but it has a long telescope.

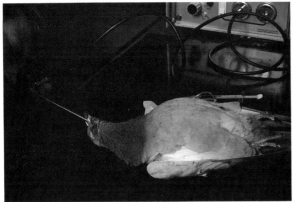

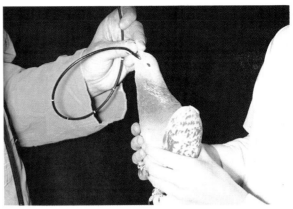

235 Bronchoscopy in a pigeon, using a rigid endoscope. Respiration can be maintained via a wide-bore needle inserted into the abdominal air sac (**237**). Anaesthesia is being maintained via a butterfly attachment in the brachial (basilic) vein.

236 Examination of the alimentary tract. Flexible endoscopes can also be used in birds. Although particularly valuable for bronchoscopy, they can, as in this picture, aid examination of the alimentary tract.

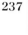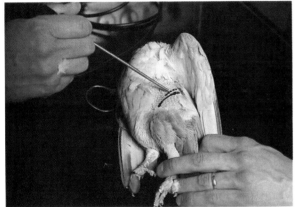

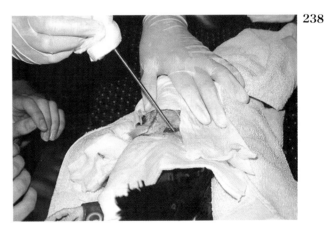

237 Laparoscopy (coeloscopy) in birds is often carried out from the left side, but various routes can be used (see p. 100). In this case, the iliotibialis cranialis muscle is marked with a continuous black line, and the last rib with a broken line. The site of insertion of the telescope is between the penultimate and final rib. This is also the position in which a needle can be inserted prior to bronchoscopy (**235**).

238 Laparoscopy in a black kite (*Milvus migrans*). Note the surgical incision on the left side. In this case a cannula has not been used.

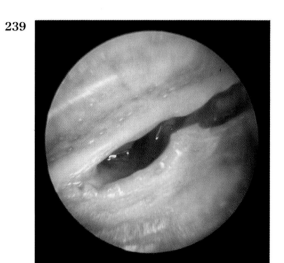

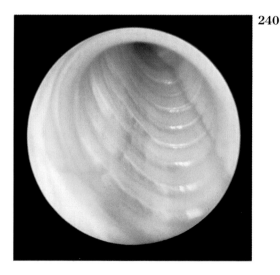

239 Palate of a European kestrel (*Falco tinnunculus*). A caseous yellow lesion due to *Trichomonas gallinae* can be seen.

240 Normal trachea of a buzzard (*Buteo buteo*).

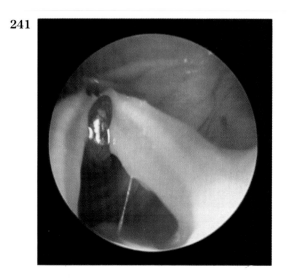

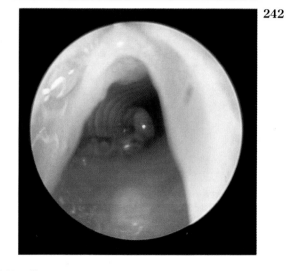

241 Glottis of a kestrel. A gapeworm (*Syngamus trachea*) can be seen protruding.

242 Gapeworm in the trachea of a kestrel.

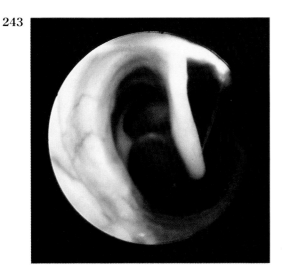

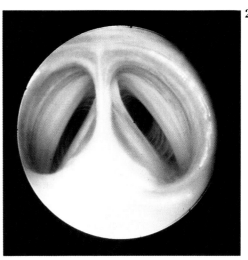

243 Normal syrinx of an eagle owl (*Bubo* sp.). The syrinx lies at the junction between the trachea and the left and right primary bronchi.

244 Syringeal bulla of a mallard (*Anas platyrhynchos*). In many species of waterfowl the syrinx is extensively modified and it is important to be able to distinguish normality from abnormality.

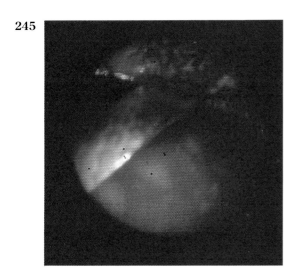

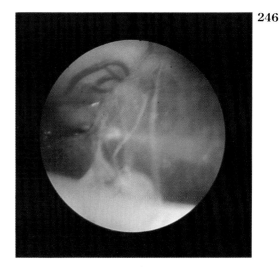

245 Spinner (fishing lure) in the stomach of a swan (*Cygnus olor*). The endoscope permits foreign bodies to be seen and, in some cases, depending upon the instrument, removed.

246 Wall of the left abdominal air sac. Note that the normal air sac is translucent, with small blood vessels: in this case there are no fat deposits.

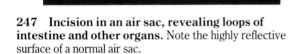

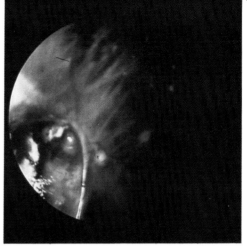

247   **Incision in an air sac, revealing loops of intestine and other organs.** Note the highly reflective surface of a normal air sac.

248   **Aspergillosis.** An early case showing distinct nodular lesions on the air sac wall. The lung is just visible (bottom left).

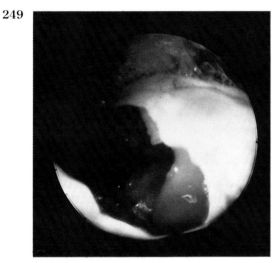

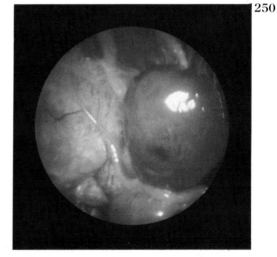

249   **Aspergillosis.** A more advanced case than that in **248**, showing extensive caseation (yellow).

250   **Anterior (cranial) area of the abdominal air sac of an immature long-eared owl (*Asio otus*).** Pale pink lung (left), red kidney (right), and adrenal and gonad (bottom centre) are visible. This is the classical view for orientation when viewing the gonads ('sexing').

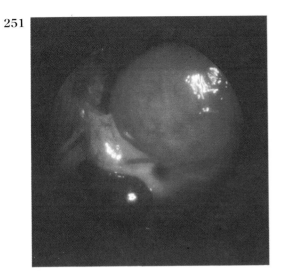

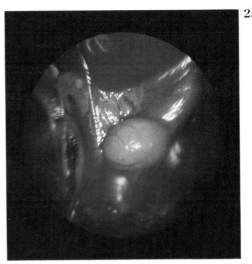

251 **One-year-old male sulphur-crested cockatoo (*Cacatua galerita*).** Note the position of the pigmented, immature testis. It is a characteristic feature of most immature cockatoos that the gonads are located ventral to the adrenal gland.

252 **Raven (*Corvus corax*) showing kidney, adrenal gland (pink) and testis (yellow).**

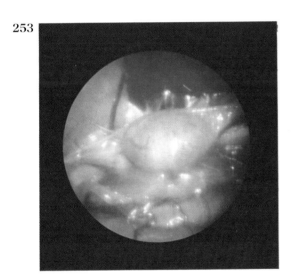

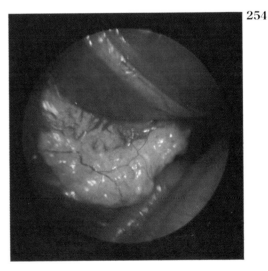

253 **Immature testis in a nine-month-old Manchurian crane (*Grus japonensis*).** Note the characteristic green colour of the immature testis in a crane.

254 **Common buzzard.** From top to bottom — kidney, adrenal gland, ovary (with small follicles) and small intestine.

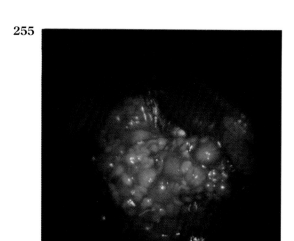

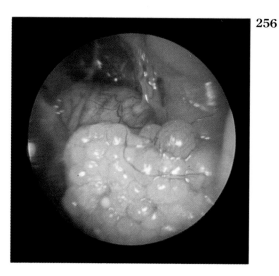

255 Ovary of an adult demoiselle crane (*Anthropoides virgo*). There are no large follicles present.

256 Common buzzard. Ovary with developing follicles and adrenal gland.

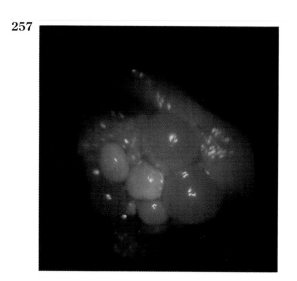

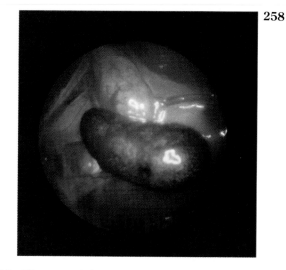

257 Common buzzard. Ovary with mature follicles.

258 Pigmented, inactive testis of an adult sulphur-crested cockatoo. Maturity can be deduced from the shape and vascularity, inactivity from the colour. An active, functional and mature testis is usually white-yellow.

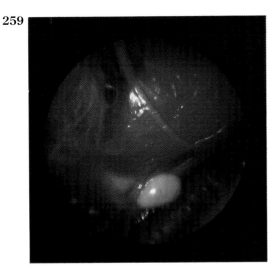

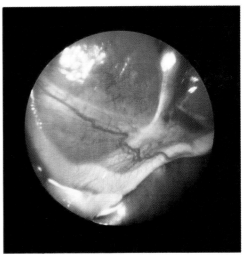

259 Raven. Kidney (top right) and testis (yellow). On the left is the septum, which separates the abdominal air sac from the cranial thoracic air sac. In this bird, there is slight inflammation of the air sac.

260 Amazon parrot (*Amazona* sp.). Kidney with ureter (bottom) packed with urates.

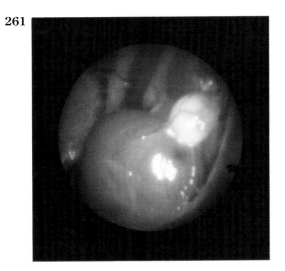

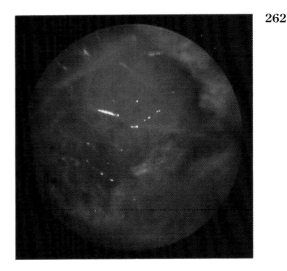

261 Cranial lobe of the kidney of an adult barn owl. There is a well-vascularised, yellow lesion, which later proved to be a neoplasm, on the dorsocaudal aspect of the lobe. The bird was clinically normal, but had a history of failing to breed. The lung is on the left.

262 Common buzzard. Pneumonia with extensive hepatisation of the lung.

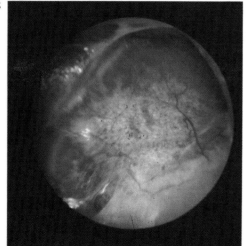

263 **Lung of eagle owl showing pneumonia with small foci of aspergillosis.**

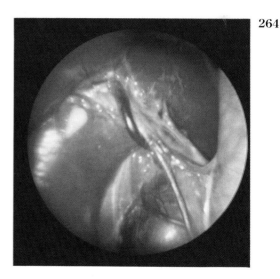

264 **Liver and gall bladder of an eagle owl.** The yellow lesion in the liver was possibly trichomoniasis.

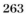

265 **Peregrine falcon (*Falco peregrinus*).** The liver, which is visible through the wall of the cranial thoracic air sac, contains foci of tuberculosis.

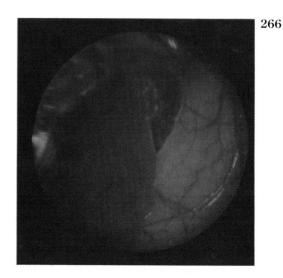

266 **Common buzzard, showing liver with small white foci and, on the right, the gizzard (ventriculus).**

267 Amazon parrot. From top to bottom – kidney, grossly enlarged spleen and the edge of the gizzard. This was possibly a case of chlamydiosis – a zoonotic disease (see pp. 13 & 114).

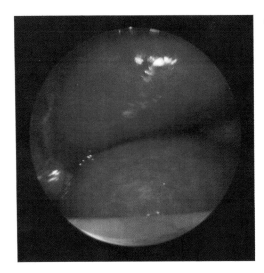

268 A student learns laparoscopy using an auriscope on a dead chicken (*Gallus domesticus*). Whenever possible, endoscopic techniques should be practised and perfected on dead animals (including postmortem specimens) or simulated models, before being carried out on live patients.

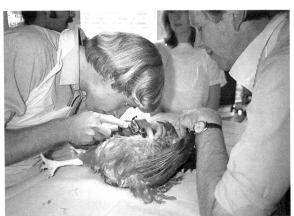

12 Endoscopy in exotic species

Most of this Atlas has dealt with the domestic dog (*Canis familiaris*) and the domestic cat (*Felis catus*), while the previous chapter concentrated on birds – an important class of vertebrate animals, in which endoscopic investigation is well established.

There are, however, many other species that may be presented for veterinary attention, and in which endoscopy can prove of value. These include a range of mammals, reptiles and amphibians. It is not the aim of this chapter to discuss and illustrate all of them in detail, but instead, to draw attention to the ways in which endoscopy can be performed and to its value in differential diagnosis and treatment.

Both rigid and flexible endoscopy can be used in non-domesticated ('exotic') species. To date, there is no comprehensive text on endoscopy in non-domesticated animals, although a number of papers have been published.

The main indications for performing endoscopy in exotic animals are summarised in **Table 1**.

Table 1	Indications for endoscopic examination in exotic species	
Indication	**Examples**	**Comments**
• Diagnosis of disease.	Foreign bodies in alimentary tract. Parasites in respiratory tract.	Endoscopy should follow a thorough clinical examination.
• Treatment of disease.	Removal of foreign bodies. Cauterisation of neoplasms.	Performed as in domesticated animals.
• Sexing of monomorphic species.	Laparoscopy in birds, reptiles and amphibians. Cloacoscopy in certain birds.	Insufflation is necessary in most reptiles and amphibians, but not in birds. Endoscopic sex determination should only be carried out when non-invasive methods have failed.
• Assessment of organ function.	Observation of gonads to determine whether gametogenesis is occurring. Monitoring of other organs to assess healing.	An important and valuable use of the endoscope, especially in captive breeding programmes.
• Facilitating other procedures.	Intubation (location of glottis). Implantation of telemetry equipment within body cavity.	Endoscopes help to illuminate and visualise external and internal structures. Magnification may be helpful.

Endoscopic appearances in 'exotic' species do not differ markedly from those in dogs, cats and other domesticated animals. Where problems arise, they usually relate to the different anatomy of the various vertebrate classes, or to the clinician's lack of familiarity with methods of restraint or anaesthesia. The latter is outside the scope of this Atlas, but the different anatomical features are important and relevant; they are therefore summarised in **Table 2** (p. 112).

Table 2	Anatomical features of relevance to endoscopy	
Class	**Features**	**Comments**
Mammalia	Presence of epiglottis.	May hamper tracheoscopy. Laryngospasm occurs in some species.
	Os penis in certain families e.g., Canidae and Mustelidae.	Usually prevents passage of a rigid endoscope *per urethram*.
Aves	No epiglottis.	Faciltates tracheoscopy, but the glottis is capable of spasm.
	Presence of syrinx.	Sometimes prevents bronchoscopy. Highly modified in some birds: may appear pathological.
	Air sacs.	Insufflation is not necessary. Air sac puncture can be used to enable ventilation to continue during tracheoscopy/bronchoscopy.
	A crop in some species.	Crop easily examined during oesophagoscopy with a rigid or flexible endoscope. The crop is a diverticulum and as such may hamper gastroscopy.
	Presence of proventriculus with no cardiac sphincter.	Facilitates examination of the stomach.
	Presence of cloaca.	Permits access to the rectum and urinary and reproductive openings.
Reptilia	No epiglottis	See above.
	Air sac and extensive ribcage in snakes.	Insufflation is not always necessary.
	Thin, sac-like lung in many species.	Care must be taken to avoid puncturing the lung.
	Long, relatively straight, gastrointestinal tract.	Facilitates examination of the upper and lower alimentary tract.
	Cloaca in some species.	See above.
	Scales and, in chelonians, a bony exterior ('shell').	Reduces access to body.
Amphibia	No epiglottis.	See above.
	Relatively thin mucous skin.	Prone to damage during examination and to desiccation/dehydration following surgery.

An important biological difference that can be relevant is that mammals (and birds) are endothermic (warm-blooded), while reptiles and amphibians are ectothermic (cold-blooded). This has a particular significance for anaesthesia, but it also means that some reptiles and amphibians need a substantial amount of time for surgical wounds to heal. Endoscopy in such species has much to commend it, if it means that surgical intervention can be minimised.

Endoscopy in exotic animals is carried out, as in other species, to investigate:

- Natural external orifices.

- The body cavity (laparoscopy).

Natural orifices

Examples are given in **Table 3**. The same general rules apply as in domesticated mammals.

Table 3	Endoscopy via natural orifices		
Orifice	**Permits examination of:**	**Groups of animal**	**Comments**
Mouth	Buccal cavity	All	Insufflation is not necessary.
	Pharynx	All	
	Oesophagus	All	Slight insufflation may prove helpful.
	Crop	Birds	
	Stomach	Many (depends on species)	The proventriculus and gizzard of birds are usually readily examined.
	Glottis	All	Generally only possible under anaesthesia. In certain mammals and some birds, spasm is a potential danger.
	Trachea/bronchi	All	
	Syrinx	Birds	
Nares	Nasal cavity and turbinate bones	Many (depends on species)	The anatomy of the nares varies. In some species endoscopy is impossible, in others only very narrow instruments can be used.
Auditory canal	Ear canal and tympanic membrane	All	The external auditory meatus of birds can be difficult to find. Most reptiles and amphibians have no canal and the tympanic membrane is readily visible from the exterior.
Anus	Rectum	Mammals and Amphibians	Remove faeces beforehand.
Cloaca	Rectum	Birds and Reptiles	Cloacal examination provides an opportunity to investigate various apertures, as well as the cloacal wall itself. It is wise to remove faeces beforehand.
	Oviduct(s)		
	Vasa deferentia		
	Internal wall of cloaca		
Vulva	Vagina	Mammals	Standard techniques can be used in both domesticated and non-domesticated species.
	Urethra	Mammals	
	Cervix	Mammals	
	Bladder	Mammals	
Penis	Urethra	Certain	Usually not possible to visualise bladder of male in species that have an os penis (mainly carnivores).
	Bladder	Mammals	

Body cavity (laparoscopy)

Some of the more important laparoscopic techniques in exotic animals are given in **Table 4**.

Table 4	Some methods of laparoscopy in exotic animals		
Group	**Entry site**	**Insufflation necessary**	**Comments**
Mammals	Lateral or central abdomen	Yes	As in dog and cat.
Birds	Sternal notch, between penultimate and last rib, or the upper part of triangle formed by the proximal femur, last rib and the cranial edge of the pubis. Other sites are possible (see p. 100).	No	The standard sites for surgical sexing. Approach is from the left side, as most birds only have a left functional ovary and oviduct.
Reptiles: Snakes	Ventral midline abdomen	Possibly	Bush (in Harrison and Wildt, 1980) prefers a paramedian approach in order to avoid blood vessels in the midline
Lizards	Ventral midline abdomen	Possibly	Avoids (paired) fat bodes.
Chelonians	Lateral (cranial) to rear leg	Usually not	Insufflation is generally contraindicated as the shell cannot expand.
Amphibians	Lateral abdomen	Yes	Only practicable in larger species.

General rules for endoscopy of exotic species

1 Handle instruments with care: some exotic species are powerful and can bite or otherwise damage delicate endoscopes.
2 Practise hygiene: like domesticated animals, exotic species are susceptible to infection, and a number can harbour organisms that may be transmissible to humans. In particular, protect surgical sites during procedures, for example, by using Op-Site™ plastic adhesive (Smith & Nephew Medical, UK), and wear protective clothing, including gloves, while performing endoscopy. Masks are not essential in every case, but should always be available. They must be worn when examining animals in which a zoonosis is suspected, e.g., chlamydiosis.
3 Do not carry out laparoscopy for sexing if other, non-invasive methods are available. However, remember that many exotic species are threatened in the world and that endoscopy for diagnostic purposes can contribute to the conservation and long-term survival of such species (both in the wild and in captivity), as well as to their welfare. In such cases, use endoscopy as an early diagnostic procedure, not a last resort.
4 Remember the particular anatomical features of exotic species which can make endoscopy difficult or different. Take every opportunity to study relevant literature beforehand. Practise on dead specimens.
5 Keep comprehensive records, not only to follow the progress of the individual patient, but also to help build up a database on endoscopic procedures (successful or otherwise) in non-domestic animals. In addition to photographs, drawings and tape-recorded descriptions can prove valuable.

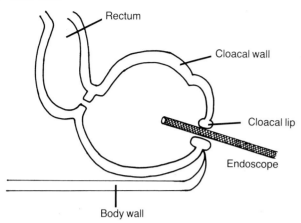

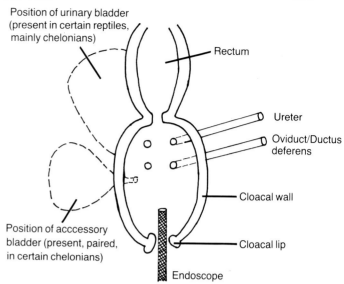

269 & 270 Diagrams of the cloaca, showing a rigid endoscope *in situ*. Note that cloacoscopy in reptiles (and birds) provides access to the rectum, and the urinary and genital orifices, as well as permitting detailed examination of the cloaca itself.

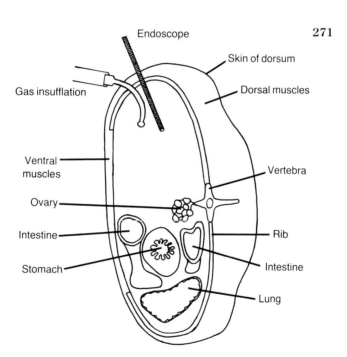

271 Diagrammatic transverse section of the body of a reptile, showing the orientation of various organs (modified from Schildger, 1987)

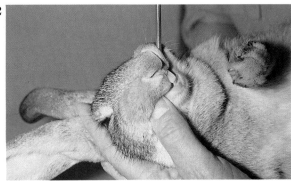

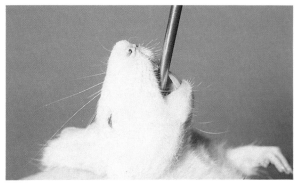

272 Examination of the buccal cavity, including the cheek, teeth and pharynx, of a rabbit (*Oryctolagus cuniculus*). Note that the animal must be properly restrained: the thumb between the lips helps to keep the mouth slightly open and facilitates viewing. Endoscopes can be inserted into the external orifices of any species. In this case a rigid instrument is being used.

273 Examination of the oesophagus of a rat (*Rattus norvegicus*). A rigid instrument can be passed down the oesophagus. This rat is being carefully held but the neck will need to be straightened if the endoscope is to pass easily over the pharynx and into the oesophagus.

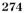

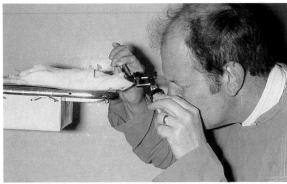

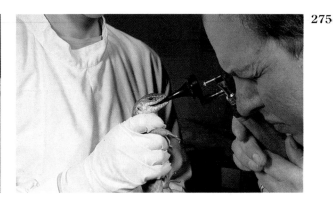

274 Examination of the glottis of a rat. A battery-operated endoscope (auriscope) provides an ideal way of locating the glottis, prior to intubation. Note that the anaesthetised animal is placed on its back to facilitate viewing of the relevant structures. The tongue is being held to one side with padded forceps.

275 Examination of the buccal cavity of a lizard (*Leiolopisma telfairii*). Similar techniques can be used in non-mammalian species. Here, an auriscope is being used to examine the buccal cavity for lesions of stomatitis. The animal is not anaesthetised. Note how it obligingly holds the speculum between its jaws!

276 Examination of the cloaca of a lizard (the same animal as shown in 275). A battery-operated instrument is used to examine the cloaca. Note how the animal is restrained. The tail must be carefully held at the base and moved dorsally to open the cloacal lips: if care is not taken, the tail may be spontaneously shed (autotomy).

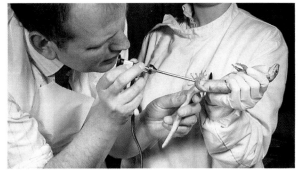

277

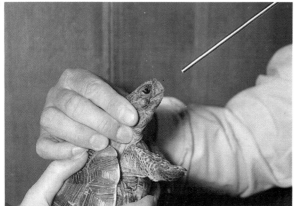

277–279 Oesophagoscopy in a tortoise (*Kinixys belliana*). The head must first be held out and the neck fully extended (**277**). The mouth must then be opened and the endoscope inserted (**278**). A finger in the corner of the jaw helps to hold the mouth open: once the endoscope is *in situ* it can be withdrawn. Finally, the endoscope is carefully passed over the tongue and down the oesophagus (**279**).

278

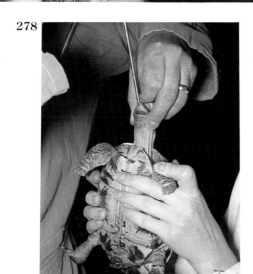

279

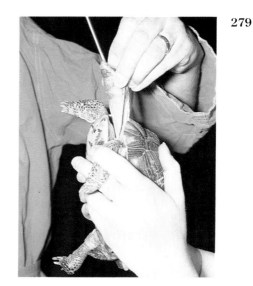

280

281

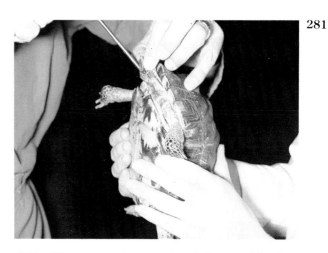

280 Cloacoscopy in a tortoise. Note how the tail is held, in this case with the fingers, thus helping to expose the cloacal opening.

281 Cloacoscopy in a tortoise. A close-up of the view in **280**.

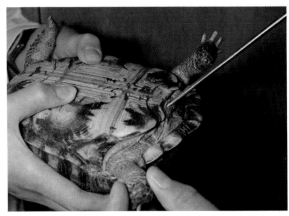

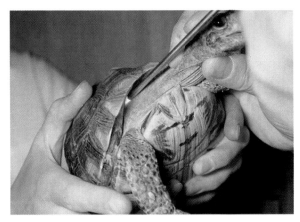

282   Cloacoscopy in a tortoise. An alternative approach is to have the tortoise on its back. However, the animal should not be kept in this position for too long.

283   Examination of the axilla of a tortoise. An endoscope also provides a useful way of detecting parasites and lesions in the axilla and other regions of chelonians that often cannot be satisfactorily examined with the naked eye. The light illuminates the area in question.

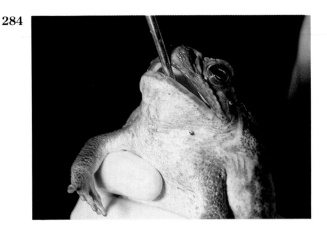

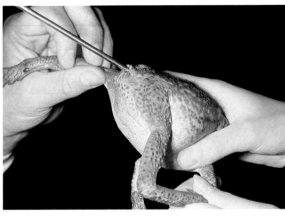

284   Pharyngoscopy and oesophagoscopy in a toad (*Bufo marinus*). Amphibians have delicate skin and mucous membranes, and must be handled very gently. Since they can also produce acrid secretions, the wearing of gloves may be wise.

285   Proctoscopy in a toad. There is usually no cloaca in amphibians, and the rectum, which is long and straight, can be examined relatively easily.

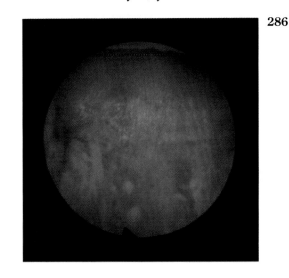

286   Endoscopic appearance of the oesophagus of a sick reptile. There is a mild hyperaemia. Changes in the appearance of the internal organs of reptiles and other 'exotic' species closely resemble those in domestic species and may, for example, include ulceration, haemorrhage and proliferative lesions.

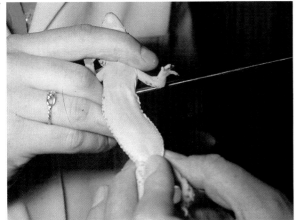

287   **Transillumination of a leopard gecko
(*Eublepharis macularius*).** Transillumination is a
technique that is underexploited in small exotic species. In
this case the patient has been taken into a darkened room
and the endoscope shone through the side of the body. The
liver and other internal organs can be seen.

288   **Transillumination of a leopard gecko.** Here,
the endoscope is being held behind the animal's body.

289   **Transillumination of a tortoise.** Another
application for transillumination is to pass the endoscope into
a hollow organ, for example, the oesophagus, and to
observe the light that is transmitted through it and the
surrounding structures. In this way, parasites and lesions
may be detected. The light can be seen glowing in the
oesophagus of this tortoise.

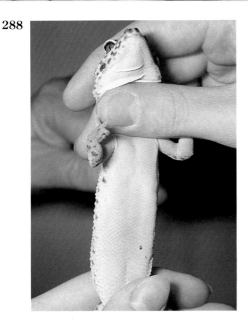

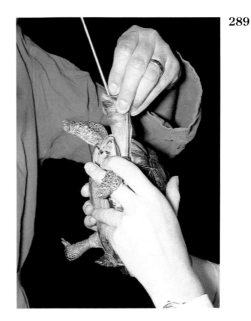

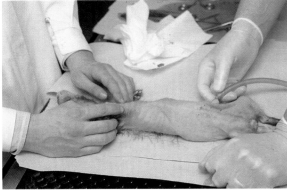

290   **Laparoscopy in a ferret (*Mustela putorius
furo*).** Laparoscopy is of great value in 'exotic' mammals. In
this case the ferret, which has alopecia, has been
anaesthetised. Gas (carbon dioxide) is being introduced into
the abdomen via a needle.

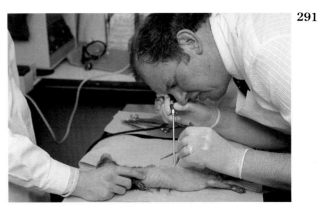

291   **Laparoscopy in a ferret.** Examination is carried
out using a rigid endoscope (in this case a human
arthroscope).

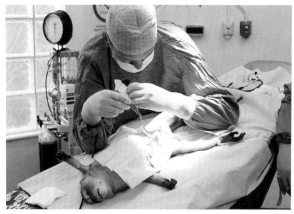

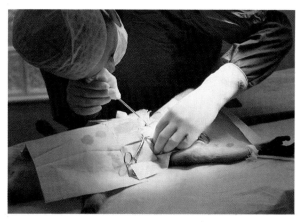

292 Laparoscopy in a monkey (*Macaca fascicularis*). Note that the operating table has been tilted so that the viscera fall forwards (towards the diaphragm), making it easier to examine the ovaries and uterus. The technique is often best performed with the endoscopist's elbows resting on the table.

293 Laparoscopy in a monkey. The use of full protective clothing is recommended when handling primates, as these animals can be a source of infection. The endoscopist's mask has been lowered only in order to prevent condensation on the eyepiece.

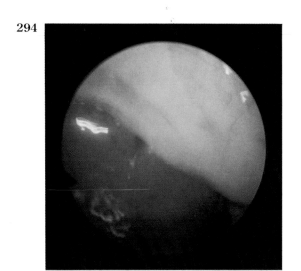

294 Laparoscopic view of the spleen and (yellow) fat in a normal monkey.

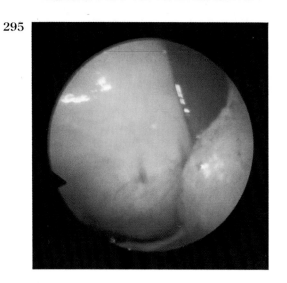

295 Laparoscopic view of the stomach in a normal monkey, with part of a lobe of liver and more abdominal fat.

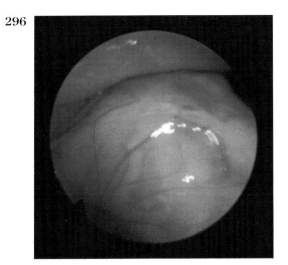

296 Laparoscopic view of a kidney, largely covered by fat, in a normal monkey. The body wall is visible at the top of the picture.

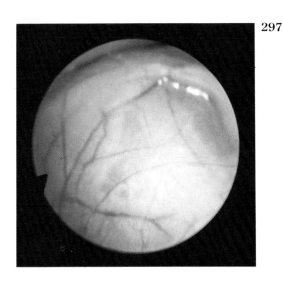

297 A closer laparoscopic view of the kidney shown in 296. The demarcation between fat and kidney is clearly visible, together with the pronounced capsular blood vessels.

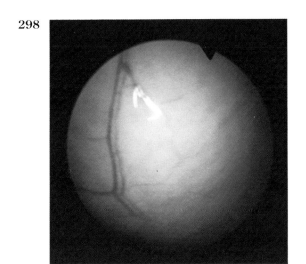

298 Serosal view of the bladder (partly distended).

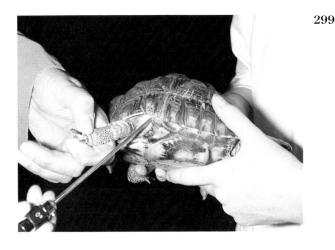

299 Laparoscopy in a tortoise. Laparoscopy (coeloscopy) can be performed in reptiles and amphibians. Here, the correct site for insertion of the rigid endoscope is shown. Insufflation is not usually required in chelonians.

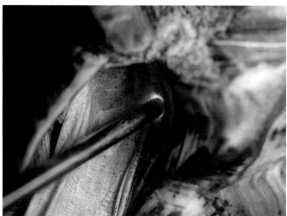

300 A closer view of the site for laparoscopy in a tortoise or other chelonians (terrapins, turtles). The alternative to this technique is to open the plastron (part of the bony 'shell').

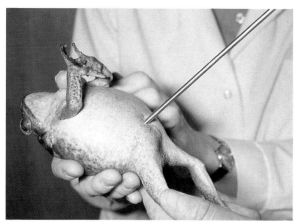

301 One possible site for laparoscopy in a toad (*Bufo marinus*). A more cranial position is hazardous as the liver may be damaged. In amphibians, insufflation is usually advisable, but because the skin is thin, great care must be taken not to overinflate and cause damage. The toad in this picture has inflated itself as part of a normal defence mechanism: this does not occur if the animal is anaesthetised.

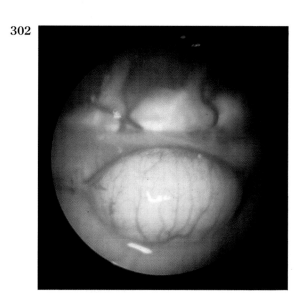

302 Laparoscopic view of a male shingle-back skink (*Trachydosaurus rugosus*), a species of lizard. The ribcage is visible at the top of the picture. The vertebral column runs from right to left. The large organ is the testis, with a paranephros on the left.

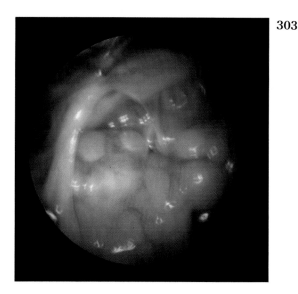

303 Laparoscopic view of a female skink (*T. rugosus*). Right and left ovaries can be seen. The vertebral column runs along the top of the picture and part of a lung is visible (bottom left).

Further reading

General texts

Jones, B. (1990). Veterinary endoscopy. *Veterinary Clinics of North America: Small Animal Practice,* **20**(5).
Keele, K.D. (1963). *The Evolution of Clinical Methods in Medicine,* Pitman Medical, London.
Miller, R.A. (1986). Endoscopic instrumentation: evolution, physical principles and clinical aspects. In *Endoscopic Surgery,* (eds) R.A. Miller and J.E.A. Wickham. *British Medical Bulletin,* **42**, 223–225.
Tams, T.R. (1990). *Small Animal Endoscopy,* C.V.Mosby, St. Louis.
Wilbush, J. (1984). Clinical information − signs, semeions and symptoms, *Journal of the Royal Society of Medicine,* **77**, 766–773.

Rhinoscopy

Böttcher, M. (1982). Rhinitis mycotica beim Hund. Diagnose und Therapie, *Tieraztliche Praxis,* **10**, 381–383.
Sullivan, M. (1987). Rhinoscopy: a diagnostic aid?, *Journal of Small Animal Practice,* **28**, 839–844.

Tracheobronchoscopy

Amis, T.C. and McKiernan, B.C. (1986). Systematic identification of endobronchial anatomy during bronchoscopy in the dog, *American Journal of Veterinary Research,* **47**, 2649–2657.
Venker-van Haagen, A.J. (1979). Bronchoscopy of the normal and abnormal canine, *Journal of the American Animal Hospital Association,* **15**, 397–410.
Venker-van Haagen, A.J. (1979). Bronchoscopy in small animal clinics: an analysis of the results of 228 bronchoscopies, *Journal of the American Animal Hospital Association,* **21**, 521–526.

Upper alimentary tract endoscopy

Happe, R.P. and van der Gaag, I. (1983). Endoscopic examination of esophagus, stomach, and duodenum in the dog, *Journal of the American Animal Hospital Association,* **19**, 197–206.
Sullivan, M. and Miller, A. (1985). Endoscopy (fibreoptic) of the oesophagus and stomach in the dog with persistent regurgitation or vomiting, *Journal of Small Animal Practice,* **26**, 369–379.

Lower alimentary tract endoscopy

Roth, L., Leib, M.S. and Monroe, W.E. (1990). Comparisons between endoscopic and histologic evaluation of the gastro-intestinal tract in dogs and cats: 75 cases (1984–1987), *Journal of the Animal Veterinary Medicine Association,* **196**, 635–638.

Vaginoscopy

Lindsay, F.E.F. (1983). The endoscopic appearance of the caudal reproductive tract of the cyclic and noncyclic bitch: post-uterine endoscopy, *Journal of Small Animal Practice,* **24**, 1–15.
Lindsay, F.E.F. and Concannon, P.W. (1986). Normal canine vaginoscopy. In *Small Animal Reproduction and Fertility* (ed) T.J. Burke, Lea and Febiger, Philadelphia.

Urethrocystoscopy

Brearley, M.J. and Cooper, J.E. (1987). The diagnosis of bladder disease in dogs by cystoscopy, *Journal of Small Animal Practice,* **28**, 75–85.
Brearley, M.J., Milroy, E.J.G. and Rickard, D. (1988). A percutaneous approach to the perineal urethra for cystoscopy in male dogs, *Research in Veterinary Science,* **44**, 380–382.
McCathy, T.C. and McDermaid, S.L. (1986). Prepubic percutaneous cystoscopy in the dog and cat, *Journal of the American Animal Hospital Association,* **22**, 213–219.
Senior, D.F. and Newman, R.C. (1986). Retrograde ureteral catheterization in female dogs, *Journal of the American Animal Hospital Association,* **22**, 831–834.

Laparoscopy

Harrison, R.M. and Wildt, D.E. (1980). (eds) *Animal Laparoscopy,* Williams & Wilkins, Baltimore.

Arthroscopy

Dandy, D.J. (1987). *Arthroscopic management of the knee* (2nd edn.), Churchill Livingstone, Edinburgh.

Kivumbi, C.W. and Bennett D. (1981). Arthroscopy of the canine stifle joint, *Veterinary Record*, **109**, 241–249.

Person, M.W. (1987). Prosthetic replacement of the cranial cruciate ligament under arthroscopic guidance, *Veterinary Surgery*, **16**, 37–43.

Person, M.W. (1989). Arthroscopic treatment of osteochondritis dissecans in the canine shoulder, *Veterinary Surgery*, **18**, 175–189.

Person, M.W. (1989). Arthroscopy of the canine coxofemoral joint, *Compendium on Continuing Education*, **11**, 930–936.

Avian endoscopy

Böttcher, M. (1981). Endoscopy of birds of prey in clinical veterinary practice. In *Recent Advances in the Study of Raptor Diseases*, (eds) J.E. Cooper and A.G. Greenwood, Chiron Publications, Keighley, pp. 101–104.

Böttcher, M. (1982a). Endoskopische Diagnostik am erkrankten Vogel, unter Einsatz möglichst schonender Methoden der Schmerzausschaltung, *Kleintier praxis*, **27**, 305–310.

Böttcher, M. (1982b). Erfahrungen mit der diagnostischen Endoskopie beim Vogel, *Tierarztliche praxis*, **10**, 183–188.

Bush, M. (1980). Laparoscopy in birds and reptiles. In *Animal Laparoscopy*, (eds) R.M. Harrison and D.E. Wildt, Williams and Wilkins, Baltimore, pp. 183–197.

Coles, B.H. (1985). *Avian Medicine and Surgery*, Blackwell Scientific, Oxford.

Cooper, J.E. (1974). Metomidate anaesthesia of some birds of prey for laparotomy and sexing, *Veterinary Record*, **94**, 437–440.

Eaton, T.M. (1988). Surgical sexing and diagnostic laparoscopy. In *Manual of Parrots, Budgerigars and other Psittacine Birds*, (ed) C.J. Price, BSAVA, Cheltenham, pp. 69–72.

Harrison, G.J. (1986). Endoscopy. In *Clinical Avian Medicine and Surgery*, (eds) G.J. Harrison and L.R. Harrison, W.B. Saunders, Philadelphia, pp. 234–244.

Jones, D.M., Samour, J.H., Knight, J.A. and Ffinch, J.M. (1984). Sex determination of monomorphic birds by fibreoptic endoscopy, *Veterinary Record* **115**, 596–598.

Kollias, G.V. (1984). Liver biopsy techniques in avian clinical practice, *Veterinary Clinics of North America: Small Animal Practice*, **14**(2), 287–298.

Kollias, G.V. (1988). Avian endoscopy. In *Exotic Animals*, (eds) E.R. Jacobson and G.V. Kollias, Churchill Livingstone, New York pp. 75–106.

Lumeij, J.T. (1988). Endoscopy. In *A Contribution to Clinical Investigative Methods for Birds, with Special Reference to the Racing Pigeon* (Columba livia domestica), University of Utrecht, pp. 152–172.

Lumeij, J.T. and Westerhof, I. (1989). Clinical endoscopy in birds, *Proceedings of 2nd European Symposium on Avian Medicine and Surgery*, Dutch Association of Avian Veterinarians, Utrecht, pp. 154–163.

McDonald, S.E. (1987). Endoscopic examination. In *Companion Bird Medicine*, (ed) E.W. Burr, Iowa State University Press, Ames, pp. 166–174.

Satterfield, W. (1980). Diagnostic laparoscopy in birds. In *Current Veterinary Therapy (VIII)*, (ed) R.W. Kirk, W.B. Saunders, Philadelphia, pp. 659–661.

Satterfield, W. (1981). Early diagnosis of avian tuberculosis by laparoscopy and liver biopsy. In *Recent Advances in the Study of Raptor Diseases*, (eds) J.E. Cooper and A.G. Greenwood, Chiron Publications, Keighley, pp. 105–106.

Endoscopy in exotic species

Brannian, R.E. (1984). A soft tissue laparotomy technique in turtles, *Journal of the American Veterinary Medical Association*, **185**, 1416–1417.

Clapp, N.K., McArthur, A.H., Carson, R.L., Henke, M.A., Peck, O.C. and Wood, J.D. (1987). Visualization and biopsy of the colon in tamarins and marmosets by endoscopy, *Laboratory Animal Science*, **37**(2), 217–219.

Cooper, J.E. (1987). Veterinary work with non-domesticated pets (III). Birds, *British Veterinary Journal*, **143**, 21–34.

Cooper, J.E. (1988). Rigid endoscopy in exotic species, In *Advances in Small Animal Practice (I)*, (ed) E.A. Chandler, Blackwell Scientific Publications, Oxford, pp. 17–29.

Cooper, J.E. and Hutchison, M.F. (1985). (eds) *Manual of Exotic Pets*, British Small Animal Veterinary Association, Cheltenham.

Coppoolse, K.J. and Zwart, P. (1985). Cloacoscopy in reptiles, *The Veterinary Quarterly*, **7**, 243–245.

Costa, D.L., Lehmann, J.R., Harold, W.M. and Drew, R.T. (1986). Transoral tracheal intubation of rodents using a fiberoptic laryngoscope, *Laboratory Animal Science*, **36**, 256–261.

Greenwood, A.G., Taylor, D.C. and Wild, D. (1978). Fibreoptic gastroscopy in dolphins, *Veterinary Record*, **102**, 495–497.

Harrison, R.M. and Wildt, D.E. (1980). (eds) *Animal Laparoscopy*, Williams & Wilkins, Baltimore.

Lumeij, J.T. and Happe, R.P. (1986). Endoscopic diagnosis and removal of gastric foreign bodies in a caiman (*Caiman crocodilus crocodilus*), *The Veterinary Quarterly*, **7**, 234–236.

Schildger, B.-J. (1987). Endoscopic sex determination in reptiles. *Proceedings of the 1st International Conference on Zoological and Avian Medicine*, Hawaii, Association of Avian Veterinarians/ American Association of Zoo Veterinarians, pp. 369–375.

Schildger, B.-J. (1989). Endoscopy for sex determination and clinical examination in reptiles. *Paper presented at the First World Congress of Herpetology*, Canterbury, September 1989.

Wrenshall, E. (1985). Laparoscopy in nonhuman primates. *Proceedings of 8th ICLAS/CALAS Symposium*, Vancouver, Gustav Fischer, Stuttgart, pp. 97–99.

Index

All references are to page numbers.
The majority of conditions affecting dogs or cats are not listed under **dog** or **cat** since all chapters, except for 11 and 12, refer exclusively to these species.